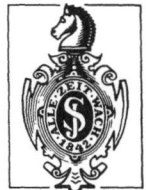

Nigel C. H. Stott

Primary Health Care

Bridging the Gap Between Theory and Practice

Foreword by John Horder

With 16 Figures

Springer-Verlag
Berlin Heidelberg New York Tokyo
1983

Nigel C. H. Stott, FRCP(Ed), MRCGP
Department of General Practice
Welsh National School of Medicine
The Health Centre, Maelfa, Llanedeyrn,
Cardiff, CF3 7PN, Wales

ISBN-13: 978-3-540-12621-8   e-ISBN: 978-1-4471-1346-1
DOI: 10.1007/978-1-4471-1346-1

Library of Congress Cataloging in Publication Data
Stott, Nigel C. H. (Nigel Clement Halley), 1939–   . Primary Health Care.
Includes bibliography and index. 1. Family medicine. I. Title DNLM: 1. Primary
Health Care. W.84.6 S888p RC46.S89 1983 362.1'0425 83-12474

The use of general descriptive names, trade marks, etc. in this publication, even if the
former are not to be taken as a sign that such names, as understood by the Trade
Marks and Merchandise Marks Act, may accordingly be used freely by anyone.

Composition by Herts Typesetting Services Limited, Hertford, England

2128/3916 543210

System, or, as Sir William Osler termed it,
the virtue of method, is the harness without which
only the horses of genius travel

Foreword

This book is about four ways of using the consultation in primary health care. One of them is very familiar, the other three a little less so. But they should all be as much a part of the repertoire of doctor or nurse as examining some system of the body or relieving pain and discomfort. If each is not used when appropriate, the full potential of the consultation is not achieved. This is the practical message of the book.

Simultaneously it is concerned with the more theoretical problems of clarifying the role of the generalist in contemporary medicine and of relating it to the wider world of people's day-to-day lives and decisions and to their interest in seeking health for their children and themselves. Is primary care too broad and general to be manageable? Is it a pot-pourri derived from other disciplines or is it distinct? If distinct, exactly how does it differ and can its principles be stated in a clear and practical way? How can it respond effectively to people's wants and needs?

The same four uses of the consultation, presented in a diagram which can be easily remembered, serve as a simple map for outlining the role of the doctor or nurse in primary care. The details of the map are filled in with clinical anecdotes and copious reference to studies from all over the world.

Thus theory runs with practice in a book which is both useful and thoughtful. The consultation, no longer confined to the problem presented, offers scope to the doctor's creative imagination working in the patient's long-term interest.

London, July 1983
John Horder, CBE, MA, BM,
BCh (Oxon), FRCP, FRGP, FRCPsych.
Visiting Fellow to the King's Fund
College, King Edward's Hospital Fund
for London
Visiting Professor at the Royal Free
Hospital, Department of Epidemiology
and General Practice

Preface

An outstanding feature of the work of the primary health care (PHC) team is its extreme generality ranging into all clinical specialty boundaries (Department of Health and Social Security 1971; The General Practitioner in Europe 1974). So broad is the base of the well-trained primary physician that few specialists would acknowledge it to be possible to have a basic grasp of so many dimensions; they are even less willing to accept that certain nurses and aides can participate responsibly in the care of a remarkable range of problems. Unfortunately, it is the few errors of the excellent and the numerically more frequent results of less competent primary care workers that are most often seen and discussed by specialists as a "second port of call", and so misconceptions about PHC are likely to continue until the newer principles and practices of PHC become more widely recognised and until the majority of those in PHC have been appropriately trained. A task which faces academics, educators and authors of PHC texts is to help to bridge the gap which still exists in the knowledge of specialists and of some generalists about the nature of modern PHC and how it is adapting to a rapidly changing world scene. The discipline of PHC has probably undergone a more rapid metamorphosis than any other in the last 30 years.

The theoretical and practical content of PHC and its associated disciplines of family medicine (Medalie 1978; Taylor 1978) and general practice (Royal College of General Practitioners 1972; Leeuwenhorst Working Party 1977) is so great and has so much overlap with other disciplines that confusion is bound to occur in the minds of students about whether this is a separate discipline or a mighty pot pourri of the component specialties. Even experienced PHC physicians sometimes fail to present the principles of their work in a succinct and practical way, and students who seem to have understood the principles of comprehensive PHC often fail to apply them in the consulting room. This rift between the theory and the practice of PHC has serious implications for teachers, patients and students and one of the purposes of this book is to show that the discipline of primary health care is beginning to achieve the unification of international principles with logical cultural diversity which are revealed in the declaration of Alma Ata (see Appendix I). Family medicine has always been in danger of becoming inappropriately esoteric or egocentric if it is provided by doctors who reject or deny the need for basic principles in their discipline and borrow from others instead. It is now in the 1980s that the emergence of important theoretical and applied principles is clearly manifest.

What are the PHC principles which are becoming internationally apparent and are these not just another game of catch-the-public by entrepreneurs? Anyone who reads this book carefully will find that the principles deal with health and ill-health and with strengthening the independence and resourcefulness of the public without removing a refuge. New insights from cross-cultural research and applications are making modern PHC a fast-moving and exciting discipline which is emerging from the wings of the academic stage and steadily establishing a remarkable role in the sociomedical arena. This monograph is written to identify some of the steps in an unusual metamorphosis and also to note some of the predators who would like to devour and absorb the evolutionary gem which, if it grows too much, could threaten their supremacy on the stage of medical progress and professional endeavour. The book is dedicated to good PHC which many powerful people are trying to embed into their own disciplines and to control before its light gets too bright. The public need and deserve primary health care which is strong enough to moderate the swinging trends of specialist intervention by the application of sound grass-root principles and ethics. Principles and ethics should be common to all professional people who work in the primary health care sector if progress is to be rooted in academic principles rather than on squabbles over the organisational surface features of the discipline.

Principles which are very simply and practically presented in the first chapters have been elaborated and presented in depth in the subsequent chapters of this book in an attempt to provide material which is graduated for junior students and postgraduates. The final chapter is really intended for advanced postgraduates because it assumes that the reader is well read.

Cardiff, 1983   Nigel C. H. Stott

References

Department of Health and Social Security (1971) The organisation of group practice. Chairman R. Harvard Davis. HMSO, London

Leeuwenhorst Working Party (1977) The work of the general practitioner. Statement by a Working Party appointed by the Second European Conference on the Teaching of General Practice. J Roy Coll Gen Pract 27:117

Medalie J (ed.) (1978) Family medicine. Williams & Wilkins, Baltimore

Royal College of General Practitioners (1972) The future of general practitioner — learning and teaching. British Medical Journal, London

Taylor R (ed.) (1978) Family medicine. Springer-Verlag, New York

The General Practitioner in Europe (1974) Second European Conference on the Teaching of General Practice. Leeuwenhorst, Netherlands

Acknowledgements

No scientific book is written without a deep debt to those whose work and wisdom are reflected in the list of references. I am grateful to them all and I hope that their work is fairly represented and acknowledged.

Many people have contributed to my work in unpublished ways: Professor R. Harvard Davis' help, counsel and friendship are greatly valued and I also acknowledge the inspiration which has come from my parents' life-work among the Zulu.

Professors B. Adams (formerly of Natal University), J. A. Strong, President of the Royal College of Physicians, Edinburgh, and G. Montgomery (formerly Professor of Pathology, Edinburgh) all kindled early research interests. Dr E. B. French and Dr R. MacNair both introduced me to the joy of clinical work in general medical practice (Edinburgh). Guy and Jan Daynes demonstrated academic mission medicine, and Dr Ronald Ingle helped me to meet Xhosa medicine men and showed me how to think in several unusual dimensions.

In Wales, my partners in the Academic Department of General Practice and the Ely Primary Care Group have all teased and tested evolving ideas and methods. Professor R. Lowe (formerly of the Department of Community Medicine at the Welsh National School of Medicine) facilitated many projects and Dr Roisin Pill has been my fellow-researcher and teacher about things anthropological.

I have been blessed by a gifted secretariat: Win Sullivan, Audrey Williams, Gloria Casseldine and Colette Trow. My wife, Mary, has suffered my distractions and assisted me in numerous ways, including a sharing of her secretarial skills. Michael Jackson of Springer-Verlag encouraged me on his periodic visits to the Welsh capital, and I am particularly grateful to Dr John Horder, Past President of the Royal College of General Practitioners, for writing a Foreword to this book.

Permission to reproduce figures was generously given by the Editor of the Journal of the Royal College of General Practitioners (Fig. 2.1), the Wellcome Foundation (Fig. 4.2), the Valley Trust (Fig. 4.4), and Dr M. Church (Figs. 5.3 and 5.4). Janice Hunter's artistic talent is illustrated by Figs. 3.3 and 3.4. Chapter 6 is based upon the Gale Memorial lecture delivered in Taunton by the author in 1982.

Contents

1. Meeting the Patient: Ideals and Realities

To understand the significance of another man's actions is to gain insight into his problems; to see what lies behind his conduct is perhaps to forgive it.

(Desmond Morris 1978)

We may praise communication, but in the human species non-communication might seem to be a more striking feature of our way.

(Robert Ardrey 1970)

Animal signals, whether vocal or visual, are largely innate, and so there can be no misunderstanding about their meaning. The flattening of a dog's ears means fear, the curl of his lip implies aggression. If a Gelada monkey lifts his eyebrows to reveal a yellow stripe, he is under threat. Animal signals are limited and inflexible, but they are precise and unlikely to be misconstrued (Ardrey 1970). The human animal is often unaware that his actions, gestures and expressions are telling their own clear story — they are the outward signals of inner attitudes and tensions. Man concentrates so hard on his words that he often seems to forget that the coded messages from his body can be either contradicting or confirming the words from his mouth. It is as if two languages are being spoken simultaneously: the familiar verbal messages and transmissions from the subconscious which are often visible rather than audible. Interpretation of gestures, tones, postures and behaviour is like translating a foreign language (the subconscious) into a common language.

In recent years, doctors and nurses have become increasingly aware of the significance of the dual languages they and their patients share because research has pointed to problems which can be missed or generated when "body language" and "verbal language" are contradictory or confused: the so-called double message.

Effective communication between two individuals depends partly upon the language and nonverbal messages issued by the two people and partly on a willingness to receive messages from one another. For example, poor results are inevitable if clinicians become inflexible in their consulting techniques (Byrne and Long 1976), because part of the messages issued by patients can be shut out and fall on deaf ears and blind eyes and clinics can be organised to make it difficult or impossible for the patient to share certain problems. A bustling atmosphere can make it awkward for many patients to communicate problems which they have difficulty in expressing in words: for example, many a physician has prescribed for a vague pain in neck or shoulder girdle and

1

missed or dismissed the sad eyes of the unhappy or depressed patient. The doctor or nurse may have no easy cure for the unhappiness but "to be understood" is the first step towards resolution of many problems (Cartwright and Anderson 1981). Sensitive discussion about a problem can sometimes help a patient tackle or come to terms with it, or result in clarification of a diagnosis which leads to conventional therapy (e.g. endogenous depression or hypothyroidism). Even the pain threshold is well known to be influenced by emotion, and failure to understand what a patient is saying or feeling is a potent cause of resistant symptoms (Korsch and Negrete 1972; Kleinman et al. 1978).

The medical profession has succeeded in maintaining an ethic and image of being caring and concerned for human welfare while holding on to a position of authority and moderate affluence in society. This is probably due to the fact that people have always needed healers in society to interpret, diagnose or treat ill-health — every tribe and race has had them — and a fair proportion of doctors have identified themselves with the communities they serve, entering into the lives and trials which their patients face. The proportion of doctors who have withdrawn from this close communication with their patients is probably increasing as technological skills have displaced the caring role and as society has valued technological skills more and more. The same society does, however, grumble about doctors who fail to understand their patients' real problems and social scientists have been quick to point to doctors' failings (Kleinman et al. 1978).

One manifestation of this duality in medical care is that analyses of the primary consultation between doctor and patient have shown that about 75% of British general practitioners use rather tightly controlled interviewing methods in their practices, about 25% using the more "open" techniques (Byrne and Long 1976). The latter group is reported to provide more openings for the patient to participate in the consultation with freer exchange of verbal and nonverbal (body-coded) messages. Numerous research workers (Korsch and Negrete 1972; Byrne and Long 1976; Johnston 1976; Engel 1977; Kleinman et al. 1978; Macquire et al. 1978; Knox et al. 1979; Verby et al. 1979; Goldberg et al. 1980; Cartwright and Anderson 1981; Zola 1981), have discovered, confirmed or amplified aspects of this work on the consultation,

Table 1.1. Consulting with barriers (examples of closed methods)

1) Little or no time spent on introduction or greeting as the patient enters
2) The posture of the consultation is formal. Clinician may be separated from the patient by a desk or the whole consultation is conducted standing (as in a busy peripheral clinic) or lying (as in a busy antenatal clinic), the clinician sometimes arriving after the patient has been undressed/prepared by an aide
3) The clinician asks questions, the patient answers. Little or no encouragement for patient to initiate comments or question
4) The clinician's manner is brisk and eye-to-eye contact with the patient is minimal (although in some cultures this is considered to be good manners)
5) Emotional reactions in the patient are soothed ("there, there") or ignored or left to nurses
6) The atmosphere in and around the consulting area is of bustle and haste. Receptionists, nurses and aides often reinforce the feeling of pressure
7) Consultations are usually terminated by the doctor with a prescription or some diagnostic advice or a procedure. The patient is hardly involved in the decisions
8) The consultation pattern and pace tend to be repetitive with little flexibility of technique from patient to patient

Table 1.2. Consulting with open methods

1) The clinician greets the patient (often by name) and preferably with warmth, e.g. "Good morning, Mrs X . . ."

2) The seating arrangement for the interview is informal, e.g. across the corner of a table if this is culturally appropriate

3) Use of social signals which encourage the patient to describe the problem without direct questioning: e.g. sufficient eye contact and nods or encouraging noises help the "history" quickly and accurately with minimal interruption

4) Clarification by (a) observation (rather than questions): e.g. "You seem to be saying that the pain moves about . . ."
   or
   "I'm still a bit confused about what the pain really stops you from doing . . ."
   (b) repeating the last word or phrase the patient said: this often encourages the patient to clarify the issue spontaneously without further questions
   (c) allowing pauses (silences) to give opportunities for the shy, or insecure, to make comments

5) Interpretation of the patient's gait, posture, gestures and facial expressions (body language): e.g. "The tears are not far away . . ."
   or
   "You seem to be dissatisfied with what you have heard . . ."

6) The atmosphere in the consultation is calm and attentive but not slow or indulgent. Time is allocated to discussion about reasons for advice or treatment or investigation

7) Most consultations finish by mutual agreement, between clinician and patient, that the task is complete

8) The consulting pattern and pace vary greatly from patient to patient

and in Tables 1.1 and 1.2 this work is summarised into practical statements to let the reader make easy comparisons between two extremes of interviewing in primary health care (PHC). The student of consulting behaviour should always try to place observed clinical encounters on a linear scale, with these two types representing opposite extremes because this discipline will emphasise the great variation which occurs between two polar types. There is some evidence that the most successful interviewers are the most flexible ones who vary the pace and comment of individual consultations substantially (Byrne and Long 1976; Fig. 1.1).

In attempting to summarise information about so complex and important a subject as interviewing, there is a danger of oversimplification and misunderstandings. It must be emphasised that the two tables are lists of examples at the extremes of consulting techniques, with all manner of variation between them, but they do serve to illustrate some salient points and the two stereotypes approximating the poles of the variation described by Byrne and Long in their analysis of general practitioners' consultations. Byrne and Long insist that they can pass no value judgements on the "right or wrong way" in clinical behaviour, but the reader is not left in any doubt that the authors' personal preference is for the more open approach. A thorough understanding of the skills involved in interviewing should, however, help the clinician to adapt his methods to different patients in different circumstances.

Cartwright and Anderson's national samples of patients in England and Wales showed that between 1964 and 1977, patients had developed higher expectations of their PHC doctors and that they were becoming much more willing to be critical; nevertheless, 90% of the 1977 sample were satisfied or very satisfied with their care and 80% regarded their doctor as easy to talk to

3

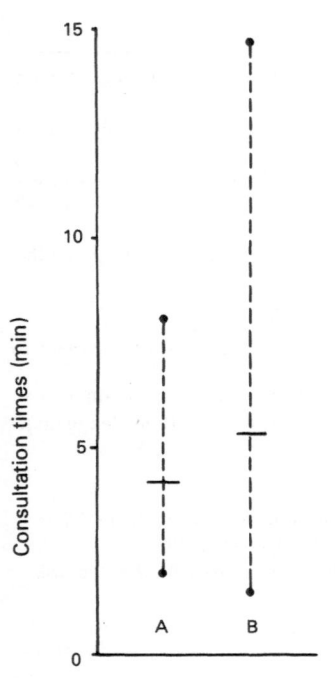

A = Malfunctioning interview
Mean 4.14 Range 2.10–8.20
Variance 1.89

B = Functioning interview
Mean 5.31 Range 1.55–14.80
Variance 6.92

Consultation time and functions

Fig. 1.1. Note the wider variation in consultation times for doctors in Group B despite comparable mean consultation time (Byrne and Long 1976).

(Cartwright and Anderson 1981). There is, however, no room for complacency because other studies which explored the issue in greater depth have suggested that people's main concerns about their illnesses are not elicited by a high proportion of doctors and nurses (Korsch and Negrete 1972; Johnston 1976; Engel 1977; Kleinman et al. 1978). Even senior medical students are reported to be less sensitive to the patients' problems than those in their first year (Knox et al. 1979), but appropriate teaching has been shown to help students and doctors to use more open techniques (Macquire et al. 1978; Verby et al. 1979; Goldberg et al. 1980).

Patients have an almost universal desire for their medical adviser of first contact to be "someone they feel they can talk to" (Hinton 1972; Stimson and Webb 1975; Byrne and Long 1976; Doyle and Ware 1977; Cartwright 1979; Fitton and Acheson 1979; Bowling 1981; Cartwright and Anderson 1981; Zola 1981). Technical skills, clinical facilities, qualifications, continuity, accessibility and status are usually considered to be less important than the way the clinician conducts himself and a consulting atmosphere which provides the patient with space and confidence to share fears and to discuss the diagnosis and treatment. It is hardly surprising that the perceptive Osler used to exhort his students to "listen to the patient, who is telling you the diagnosis".

4

The consensus from most published work is that doctors who practise with more open interview techniques have the best opportunities to hear what the patient is saying. Whether the clinician is then able to use the information collected will depend on appropriate training in clinical skills and in the skills of effective communication, because most clinical successes and educational successes depend on patient participation and co-operation — issues which are dealt with in more detail in subsequent chapters.

Reasons for Consulting Patterns

The dominance of more closed techniques in consulting sessions is unlikely to be a quirk of the European culture in which much of the quoted research was conducted because people who have worked in the front lines of modern primary health care in various parts of the world recognise similar trends (Zola 1981). A possible exception to this rule is the protected affluence of private practice where it is widely acknowledged that patients pay for time, convenience and sometimes even for common courtesy. In parts of the world where nurses or aides play a large part in the delivery of primary health care, they too are capable of adopting closed consulting tactics, perhaps because the doctors are often their teachers or supervisors; perhaps because circumstances force this pattern upon them?

To understand these trends towards more closed consultation techniques it is necessary to consider factors which may influence clinicians to work in this way.

1) Educational influences.
2) Cultural and social factors.
3) Pressure of work.
4) Authority and cover-up.

1) Educational Influences

The first impact of education on the future performance of doctors and nurses is the selection process which allows certain individuals to enter these disciplines. A system which draws in those with exceptional intellectual abilities may not be best at selecting those with patience and a genuine interest in their fellow men. Objective information on this point is difficult to obtain but research methods which permit an assessment of an individual's personality in terms of warmth, genuineness and empathy (Truax and Mitchell 1971; Diseker and Michielutte 1981), could prove to be of more relevance to meeting future patients' needs than first-class school results. In one study of medical students their empathy, measured on the Hogan scale, was negatively correlated with entrance examination results (Diseker and Michielutte 1981).

The formal teaching of interviewing skills is a very recent development in medical schools and so most doctors and nurses have had little or no training in this subject and many even resent the suggestion that interviewing may differ from conventional clinical history taking. A result of such attitudes is that students are still exposed to many teachers who are full of antipathy to the recent developments and some are not pleased by evidence that both students and doctors can be helped to achieve more effective and active interviewing skills in their clinical work (Peck 1978; Knox et al. 1979; Verby et al. 1979).

Students are usually introduced to their first patients by being shown physical signs or by being given the name of a patient to interview on the ward. The first few weeks of interviewing experience are frightening if the student is to avoid feeling stupid because the emphasis from those most highly differentiated of all doctors — the teaching hospital specialists — is biased heavily towards finding a diagnostic answer. Understanding the individual is a rather different process with very different skills and values, so it comes as no surprise that a high proportion of doctors never adapt their interview methods from the mechanistic techniques they are taught (Stimson and Webb 1975; Byrne and Long 1976).

Unfortunately, the clinician who is blind to or unprepared for the more delicate aspects of communication is unlikely to perceive his weaknesses and can continue for years to ride rough-shod over the very issues the patients are most concerned about, particularly when problems are multiple or couched in indirect language or cultural diversity. For example, fertility is an immensely important virtue to most Zulu maidens and this cultural imperative can make the interpretation of "abdominal pain" rather difficult for a doctor who has taken a thorough but unhelpful traditional clinical history but failed to interpret his patient's sad and sagging posture — the notes which read "Para 0 + 0", "unmarried" and "ill-defined abdominal pain" being a marker of the doctor's failure to interpret both cultural mores and the patient's posture and mood. Another example would be British medical students who sit with a general practitioner teacher and diagnose "upper respiratory infections" or "otitis media" with confident ease yet often fail to notice that an otherwise relatively healthy child has been brought by a mother or father who was looking unduly anxious or worn. Under the circumstances, the traditional prescription becomes nothing more than an outward and visible sign of the student's inability to identify the other problems as perceived or felt by the parent.

Fortunately, more and more teachers in primary health care are becoming familiar with the need to help their students discover the skills involved in successful interviewing, but the teaching time that most medical schools are able to allocate to such activities in their curricula remains limited and the situation is unlikely to change until specialists start to value and express more approval of the PHC teaching programmes in their own schools of medicine.

2) Cultural and Social Factors

Alien languages, dialects and accents are powerful influences in causing the separation of subgroups in our society and the growth of poor communication and misunderstandings which in turn lead to a lack of compassion and to estrangement. Ardrey (1970) argues that this creation of strangers is a biological reality which the human animal shares with other animals to protect one subgroup from exploitation by another and he is pessimistic about the possibility of genuine understanding across cultural barriers. Few doctors or nurses would accept such pessimism or that their interview methods sometimes make life difficult for patients whose linguistic background is foreign, but there is no doubt that cross-cultural consultations can be very time consuming. Evidence that Asian-trained doctors in British general practice are less prepared to be tolerant of minor emotional and less severe illnesses than British-trained doctors points to the same problem (Cartwright and Anderson 1981).

Another factor which modifies the performance of PHC consultations is social class: the working classes tending to have shorter consultations and fewer explanations from their doctors than those patients of professional and managerial classes, a trend which is constant when either complex or simple diagnoses are made (Pendleton and Bochner 1980). That there is insufficient sharing of information by physicians with their patients is born out in a much larger study (Byrne and Long 1976), and this is a well-reported source of irritation to patients (Waitzkin and Stoeckle 1972; Stimson and Webb 1975; Fitton and Acheson 1979). A national survey in the United Kingdom in 1964 showed that 75% of the population wanted their physicians to share more information about their problems. About 10 years later the figure had risen to 85% (Cartwright and Anderson 1981), illustrating the increasing numbers of patients of all social classes who want to know the nature and cause of their illness, the results of investigations and how treatment is progressing. They are less and less prepared "to leave it to the doctor".

In some parts of the world, patients may appear to accept authoritarian clinical handling — perhaps because they have no choice — but this does not remove their need for involvement in their own care and the beneficial effect that involvement can have upon compliance with treatment or health education (Korsch and Negrete 1972; Haynes 1976; Diseker and Michielutte 1981; Zola 1981). Patients can be involved in two major ways:

a) by ascertaining and taking seriously their beliefs and concerns about the problem (Becker 1979);
b) by encouraging participation in all the decisions which are made about their health (Krantz 1980).

Does nonverbal body language have different forms in different cultures? A dictionary of sign language in many cultures demonstrated that many culturally specific signals do occur (Brun 1969), for example shaking hands can be warm in the West or insulting to some Asians and a nod of the head does not mean "yes" in all races. Even eye-to-eye contact can be used or abused according to local custom and whether a woman or man is involved. Shifty attitudes and humble respect can be easily confused without knowledge of local cultural mores. Many colourful examples of such differences can be found in Morris' (1978) richly illustrated *Manwatching* and the PHC doctor or nurse who is working in a foreign culture would do well to make a serious attempt to learn both verbal and nonverbal languages of the local people. Those who work in multiracial areas have a particularly difficult task on their hands if they are to communicate with their patients and involve them in their health care, particularly as the ethnocentric communities or family groupings tend to be most suspicious of medical care (Suchman 1964).

Total dependence on interpreters is an alternative solution to the dilemma of cultural diversity but another, less acceptable, solution is often applied in casualty departments or the less sensitive corners of medical care: the practice of veterinary-type medicine on alien human beings, in which most verbal and nonverbal messages are disregarded in favour of pure physical diagnosis. The patient is reduced to being a stranger in the medical machine, acceptable (perhaps) for an uncomplicated laceration but an unhappy experience for those who have the fears or misunderstandings or grievings to which human beings are subject.

3) Pressure of Work

When you get to the doctor he lifts his pen to the pad before you say a thing . . . you are lucky if you 'ave time to sit down before he has finished. (Welsh miner's wife)

Too much time makes you slow down — a full waiting area takes as long to deal with as when it is half empty when you begin . . . (English doctor)

I saw one hundred patients today — like a black puddin' factor it was . . . (Scottish doctor in rural Africa)

Tomorrow is another day . . . I'm off to bed and sixty are still sleeping outside the out-patient department. (Zulu doctor in urban hospital)

Comments like these reflect feelings about pressure of clinical work in a way which statistics cannot convey. Similar sentiments could have been expressed in large antenatal clinics, casualty departments, busy mission hospitals, peripheral clinics and other PHC locations all over the world where doctors, nurses and aides feel besieged by patients.

One of the interesting features about very busy working conditions is that many doctors and nurses become proud of their pace of work, as if the hallmark of PHC success is speed. Cartwright (1979) — a social scientist — was shocked to find that most general practitioner consultations were conducted in less than 5 minutes, yet a well-quoted classic entitled *Six minutes for the patient* (Hopkins 1973) has done much to provide an aura of respectability for the brief consultation by encouraging it to be seen as one episode in a sequence of continuing contacts, rather than as an isolated event.

The eighteenth-century surgeon felt similar pride when his dexterity with the knife was being judged in "seconds on the job" rather than by the clinical result because in the pre-anaesthetic era, pain and survival of the patient were inversely related to the duration of the operation. Until the discovery of anaesthetics, the need for haste must have been a major barrier to the development of modern surgical techniques. The analogy can be carried further as scientific advances have increased the range of skills and equipment in PHC at an unprecedented rate. Opportunities for prevention, care and cure have proliferated for ambulant patients and the pressure for innovation and changes of working methods is rising constantly. Under these circumstances, speed of work is a necessity and also a barrier to having sufficient time for reorganisation and a resetting of ideas and ideals.

The advent of delegation and sharing of many duties with nonmedical staff has been one of the great milestones in PHC during the last two decades but there has been considerable resistance from some medical and nursing sectors (Bowling 1981). The creation of a PHC team is not always easy because the generalist doctor and nurse have fewer clearly demarcated boundaries to their work than specialists and an overlap of skills is a potential source of uncertainty and friction between PHC team members. Legal matters in an increasingly litigation-minded world pour fuel on this issue. Nevertheless, many PHC teams can operate successfully (Department of Health and Social Security 1971; Marsh and Kaim Caudle 1976; Ruben et al. 1978), and greater delegation of duties by doctors and nurses is a potential source of time. This provides hope for a shift away from the prevailing "speedy work" ethos of PHC and the provision of time for every doctor to reconsider interview methods and perhaps for more patients to feel that they have a doctor who understands their problem(s). Whether the advent of team-work and delegation to PHC will lead to as great a revolution in methods as the impact of anaesthesia on surgeons remains to be seen, as both doctors and nurses are often reluctant delegators (Bowling 1981) and more time does not necessarily lead to more skilled consultations unless the people involved also develop greater awareness of patients' needs for involvement in the clinical process (Byrne and Long 1976). Individual beliefs and fears should be handled as effectively as a tonsillitis but the skills are very different.

4) Authority and Cover-up

Doctors say some extraordinary things to their patients and no doubt other, less studied, members of the health professions would also qualify for such comment if a tape recorder was planted in their consulting rooms. For example:

Don't argue with me, I'm the doctor and you are the patient. You will do as I say or go.

The intensity of this doctor's feelings suggests a serious threat to his self-esteem and authority. The patient is left with Hobson's choice: to submit or fight back, but it is unlikely that either course would help much. The relationship is clear "the doctor has absolute authority or else . . .".

A reluctance to negotiate with patients by sharing information about certainties and uncertainties is also witnessed in other branches of medicine, as the following exchanges illustrate:

Patient:	(to her family doctor): "I have just had my second out-patient appointment with Mr X. (Neurosurgeon) for my headaches" (caused by trigeminal neuralgia).
Family doctor:	"Yes . . ."
Patient:	"He behaved very oddly" (giggles).
Family doctor:	"Oh?"
Patient:	"I sat in his room after waiting 2 hours and he looked up and said: 'Do you want the nerve to your face cut? Tell me yes or no!' I started to say 'But is that necessary' and he interrupted and said' 'No, no, you must answer my question. Tell me, yes or no(!) do you want the nerve cut?'."
Family doctor:	"What did you say?"
Patient:	"I said 'no' because I could see that he was in no mood to talk to me . . . you see doctor, the pain has been improving a little but it is a nuisance . . . what do you think I should do?"

The striking thing about this account was the patient's good-humoured tolerance of the surgeon's high-handed attitude. She bore him no malice but she did need help to come to a decision about the meaning and likely duration of her symptoms. She said as she left: "I feel that the nerve is gradually healing."

A doctor, or nurse or aide or receptionist, has authority over the patient by virtue of training or position and many patients feel vulnerable, particularly in the hospital environment. The authority of the ward sister has been caricatured in innumerable anecdotes, stories and jokes, and both medical students and pupil nurses will recall their awe of some colourful matron or sister. What chance have patients for self-assertion and expression in such an environment and what chance have the students of emerging from such a milieu with anything other than authoritarian models of professional behaviour?

Tears, anger, doubt and questions are often upsetting to medical authority because human emotions cannot be handled by authoritarian methods alone. If the doctor or nurse involved is uncomfortable and unable to share the patients' feelings and interpretations, it is possible to cover up with anger, detachment or denial. McNamara (1974) showed that students experienced greatest difficulty with the same human emotions, and Knox et al. (1979) reported a great need for students to have help to learn skills necessary to handle emotional episodes constructively. When doctors or nurses can cope with their own uncertainties and accept that they all still stand on the touch-line of full clinical understanding, they will have no need to cover up doubts with dogma. Many patients want to understand and negotiate their diagnoses, treatments, prognoses and paths to health. Too few doctors and nurses are prepared to let them negotiate (Balint 1964; Browne and Freeling 1967; Stimson and Webb 1975; Byrne and Long 1976; Zigmond 1978; Cartwright and Anderson 1981; Good and Good 1981).

The single most important determinant of the outcome of any relationship is honesty. People may get away with barriers of cover-up and pretence for short periods of time but any continuing relationship can only be stable if honest communication occurs between both parties. Browne and Freeling (1967), in a typically practical manner, point out that it is common for strong feelings to be around when patient meets doctor and so misunderstanding or misinterpretation of the doctor's words and attitudes is likely unless the doctor is able to share personal attitudes with clarity and honesty.

The most successful psychotherapists are those who are warm, genuine and empathetic (Truax and Mitchell 1971), but such people are also open to abuse by their patients unless they learn to handle the clingers, the demanders, the manipulators and the rejectors (Groves 1978). The detachment and authority of the traditional clinician may diminish personal emotional involvement and pain for the price of some of the most subtle methods of communication. Nowhere is the dilemma as acute as in PHC where relationships with patients often continue for many years and mistakes are lived with, not buried or discharged; a point which will be returned to in Chapter 3, when considering continuing care, and Chapter 6, when the important "refuge principle" is analysed.

At the opposite extreme from cold and detached interviewing of patients is the overzealous exploration of every nuance and nonverbal leak of information, coupled with unnecessary probing into the recesses of patients' experiences, taboo areas and ideas of causation. This type of medical history taking can be more insensitive to people's feelings than ignoring them completely. The student or doctor who feels or teaches that a detailed history of beliefs, sexual and emotional factors in every patient is essential for effective clinical work is indulging in a crude inquisitory process which at best is ill-mannered and at worse a "rape of the mind" (Zigmond 1978).

Meeting the patient successfully and effectively demands clinical history taking which is conducted with skills which are becoming sufficiently understood to be taught effectively. Whether the students learn and apply them will be determined by attitudes in their places of work and in the communities they will serve. The indications are that the gap between the theory and practice of clinical interviewing is beginning to close but, as this happens, the debate about what is right or wrong use of consultation time will intensify and the pressure for sharing of duties and information is likely to increase.

References

Ardrey R (1970) The social contract. Collins, London

Balint M (1964) The doctor, his patient and the illness. Pitman Medical, London

Becker M (1979) Understanding patient compliance: the contributions of attitudes and other psychosocial factors. In: Cohen S (ed) New directions in patient compliance. Lexington, New York.

Bowling A (1981) Delegation in general practice. Tavistock, London

Browne K, Freeling P (1967) The doctor–patient relationship. Livingstone, London Edinburgh

Brun T (1969) The international dictionary of sign language. Wolfe, London

Byrne PS, Long BL (1976) Doctors talking to patients. A study of the verbal behaviour of general practitioners consulting in their surgeries. HMSO, London

Cartwright A (1979) Minor illness in the surgery. In: Management of minor illness. King Edward's Hospital Fund, London, pp 117–134

Cartwright A, Anderson R (1981) General practice revisited. Tavistock, London

Department of Health and Social Security (1971) The organisation of group practice. A report for the Standing Medical Advisory Committee. Chairman RH Davis. HMSO, London

Diseker RA, Michielutte R (1981) An analysis of empathy in medical students before and after clinical exposure. J Med Educ 56(12):1004–1010

Doyle BJ, Ware JE (1977) Physician conduct and other factors that affect consumer satisfaction and medical care. J Med Educ 52(10):793–801

Engel GL (1977) The need for a new medical model: a challenge for biomedicine. Science 196:129–136

Fitton F, Acheson HWK (1979) Doctor/patient relationship. HMSO, London

Goldberg DP, Steele JJ, Smith C, Skivey L (1980) Training family doctors to recognise psychiatric illness with increased accuracy. Lancet ii: 521–523

Good BJ, Good MJD (1981) The meaning of symptoms: a cultural hermeneutic model for clinical practice. In: Eisenberg L, Kleinman A (eds) The relevance of social science for medicine. Reidel, Dordrecht Boston London, pp 165–196

Groves JE (1978) Taking care of the hateful patient. New Engl J Med 298:883–887

Haynes RB (1976) A critical review of the determinants of patient compliance with therapeutic regimes. In: Sackett DL, Haynes RB (eds) Compliance with therapeutic regimes. Johns Hopkins University Press, Baltimore pp 26–39

Hinton K (1972) Dying, 2nd edn. Pelican, London, pp 134–135

Hopkins P (1973) The time factor. In: Balint E, Norrell JS (eds) Six minutes for the patient: interaction in general practice. Tavistock, London, pp 142–153

Johnston M (1976) Communication of patients' feelings in hospital. In: Bennett AE (ed) Communication between doctors and patients. Nuffield Provincial Hospital Trust/Oxford University Press, Oxford, pp 31–45

Kleinman AM, Eisenberg L, Good B (1978) Culture, illness and care. Ann Int Med 88:251–258

Knox JDE, Alexander DW, Manson AT, Bennett A (1979) Communication skills and undergraduate medical education. Med Educ 13:345–348

Korsch RM, Negrete VF (1972) Doctor–patient communication. Sci Am 227(2):66

Krantz DS (1980) Assessment of preferences for self-treatment and information in health care. Journal of Personality and Social Psychology, 39:977–990

McNamara M (1974) Talking with patients: some problems met by medical students. Br J Med Educ 8:17–23

Macquire P, Rue P, Goldberg D, James S, Hyde C, O'Dowd T (1978) The value of feedback in teaching interviewing skills to medical students. Psych Med 8:695–704

Marsh GN, Kaim Caudle P (1976) Team care in general practice. Croom Helm, London

Morris D (1978) Manwatching. A field guide to human behaviour. Triad/Granada, London

Peck D (1978) Communications and compliance. Bull Brit Psych Soc 31:348–352

Pendleton DA, Bochner S (1980) The communication of medical information in general practice consultations as a function of patients' social class. Soc Sci Med 14A:669–673

Ruben MR, Fry RE, Plovnick MS (1978) Making health teams work: an educational program. In: Medalie JH (ed) Family medicine. Williams and Wilkins, Baltimore, pp 316–328

Stimson G, Webb B (1975) Going to see the doctor. Routledge & Kegan Paul, London Boston

Suchman E (1964) Sociomedical variations among ethnic groups. Social patterns of illness and medical care. Am J Soc 70:319–331

Truax CB, Mitchell KM (1971) Research on certain therapist interpersonal skills in relation to process and outcome. In: Bergin AE, Garfield SL (eds) Handbook of psychotherapy and behavioural change. John Wiley, New York, pp 299–344

Verby JE, Holden P, Davis RH (1979) Peer review of consultations in primary care: the use of audiovisual recordings. Br Med J 1:1686–1688

Waitzkin H, Stoeckle JD (1972) The communication of information about illness. Adv Psychosom Med 8:180

Zigmond D (1978) When Balinting is mind-rape. Update 1:1123–1126

Zola IK (1981) Structural constraints in the doctor–patient relationship: the case of non-compliance. In: Eisenberg L, Kleinman A (eds) The relevance of social science for medicine. Reidel, Dordrecht Boston London, pp 241–252

2. Extending the Consultation Goals

The foundations for PHC are laid in consultations with patients. Here expectations are fulfilled or dashed and here sequences of decisions and events are initiated which can be of momentous importance to the patient and family. What appears superficially trivial sometimes proves to be very serious and what is dismissed is often an opportunity missed for prevention rather than cure. No specialist has such diversity of demands and opportunities, and great professional vigilance is required if standards are to be maintained or improved in the various places where PHC is practised.

The first professional requirement for good PHC is skill at exchanging information with people — an issue which was dealt with in Chapter 1. The second, closely related, requirement should be shared with all specialists — an ability to make the patients feel that their felt needs are heard seriously, however incredible or laughable or selfish they may seem initially. The third basic requirement is adequate diagnostic and therapeutic skills to deal with the diversity of PHC problems; it is here that the principles and practices of modern PHC begin to diverge from other specialties to form their unique position as an embryonic discipline.

The Surface Anatomy of Primary Health Care

Our starting point is a simple aide-memoire to reveal the potential in every PHC consultation in a form which is easily memorised and understood by the most junior of students (Fig. 2.1). The four interrelated areas embrace many skills which the PHC clinician can use to the patients' benefit and the basis of

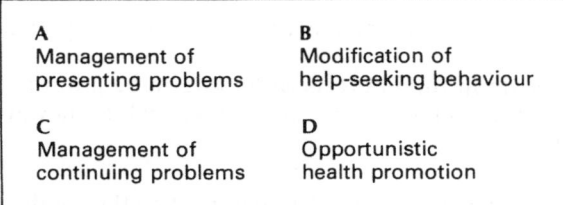

A Management of presenting problems	B Modification of help-seeking behaviour
C Management of continuing problems	D Opportunistic health promotion

Fig. 2.1. The exceptional potential in each primary care consultation — an aide-memoire (Stott and Davis 1979).

this aide-memoire is intimately related to the decisions which face every PHC clinician, whatever his or her educational background and within whatever system of care he or she operates. Junior students can learn the outline, which is subsequently elaborated by the acquisition of knowledge, skills and maturity, and postgraduates can be encouraged to consider their clinical actions against the framework (Stott and Davis 1979). It clarifies the practical implications of many of the concepts described in detailed texts and working parties (Department of Health and Social Security 1971; Royal College of General Practitioners 1972; The General Practitioner in Europe 1974; Leeuwenhorst Working Party 1977; Taylor 1978) and it also helps to demonstrate how PHC and specialist medicine should differ in many consultations.

The aims of the framework are as follows.

1) To provide a simple theoretical base from which a clinician can develop the full potential in any PHC consultation.
2) To highlight some unique features of modern PHC.
3) To provide a basis for teaching in PHC which is simple enough for the undergraduate or assistant but equally valid for the postgraduate when more detailed knowledge and skills are included in the same basic structure.
4) To allow the philosophy, principles and research achievements in PHC to be discussed within a practical patient-centred framework.

The framework (Fig. 2.1) is not a classification of knowledge, skills and attitudes. It is a synthesis of principles to reveal potential strategies which can be used in PHC in every contact with patients. Comprehensive care is a blend of the four interrelated Areas A–D and, although it is often inappropriate to work through all four areas in a consultation, it is usually unacceptable for a clinician to function at Area A level alone. The presenting problem can be diagnosed in a conventional manner but the other dimensions to the consultation will only begin to be identified and understood if the clinician also asks himself the following questions.

1) Why is this patient (or family) consulting in this way and at this time? Is the patient (or family) likely to behave in the same way next time a similar problem occurs? (Area B.)
2) What other continuing problems does this patient (or family) have which I should monitor/enquire about while they are in my consulting room or clinic? (Area C.)
3) Is it appropriate for me to take the opportunity to encourage this patient (or family):
   (a) to modify their life-style in the interests of long-term health, or
   (b) to permit me to practise a relevant screening activity while they are with me? (Area D.)

The practice of these three dimensions has a profound impact on the conduct and sequelae of the consultation in PHC and the background principles to each will be considered in greater detail in later chapters. This chapter will be used to illustrate use of the framework by doctors, nurses and aides in different cultures and situations. The simplicity of the basic concept means that a logical structure can be applied to every consultation in PHC within the limits of the skills and resources that are available. Students also become aware of what is omitted if the full PHC potential is not being realised due to personal or physical restraints. Unfortunately it is still common for some doctors to remark that most PHC work is easy or trivial. Such comments often come from the ill-informed or inexperienced, but not always. It is an unfortunate truth, as we saw in Chapter 1, that many doctors use consulting techniques which block communication with patients and there is evidence to show that many consultations still deal with the presenting problem(s) alone, little attempt being made to widen the consultation beyond Area A. Paradoxically, the analyses of consultation behaviour discussed in Chapter 1 often dwell so much on interviewing that other skills become underemphasised. Byrne and Long, for example, defined five phrases in the consultation.

    I Establishing a relationship.
   II Doctor attempts to discover the reason for the patient's attendance.
 III Doctor conducts a verbal and/or physical examination.
 IV The condition is considered (information sharing).
   V The consultation is terminated.

Each of these phrases is centred on the presenting problem(s) (Area A in Fig. 2.1) with the possible exception of phase two in which help seeking (Area B) is touched upon. The improvement of interviewing skills has been a valuable contribution to the art and science of PHC, but a clinician who fails to adapt his methods to embrace more than Area A can limit the scope of PHC and fail to appreciate the contribution of new equipment, tools, staff and facilities which can enhance the work of Areas B, C and D and lift PHC to a fresh level of professional skill and organisation and differentiate it from specialist medicine.

The potential in every consultation, including sound communication, should be a spur to those who want to work to realise better PHC and a barrier to those who are lazy or inappropriately trained for the task. Nurses, health visitors and aides who participate in modern PHC can often deal with a great number of PHC functions extremely competently and without their collaboration the task of the doctor becomes impossible or irrelevant. For too long has there been pretence that hole-in-the-wall patch-and-dash general practice bears any relationship to modern PHC, and now the newer threat of a fragmented PHC team with doctors, nurses and health visitors, social workers and others all pulling in different 'specialist' directions is equally ludicrous (Bowling 1981). The potential for a co-ordinated, and responsible approach to patient care is feasible and highly desirable, but a doctor who fails to widen most consultations beyond the presenting problems is very unlikely to discover a role in PHC teams which have a co-ordinated approach to both health and illness.

The examples which follow have been chosen to illustrate fragments of what can happen when an alert clinician begins to widen PHC to move beyond the management of presenting problems into the other three broad areas depicted

15

in Fig. 2.1. Patients' felt needs obviously have to be given a priority in all consultations, but in many PHC encounters the felt or expressed needs are really less relevant to the individual's health than other factors which the patients may have ignored, be unaware of or be struggling with silently.

Example 1: Limited Use of Framework

John P. (38 years) comes with his wife a few days after Christmas. He has had a sore throat for a week and a tender lump is now appearing on the left side of his neck. A tender lymph gland 3 cm in diameter is palpable in the deep upper cervical glands and his throat is slightly inflamed. The doctor decides to treat John P. with penicillin for an acute lymphadenitis, a possible complication of a resolving streptococcal throat infection (Area A — physical only). However, realising that John P. is less interested in the treatment than in why he should have developed the problem, the doctor encouraged him to comment . . . "I suppose I was run-down doctor . . . I have been working rather late". It is also unusual for a wife to accompany her young husband to a doctor in British society — unless she is very anxious about something (Area B — help-seeking pattern). The doctor observed: "You must be very worried about him" and she responded: "Yes, he won't tell you half of what is going on . . . ask him about the lump in his testicle."

In this example, the doctor could have functioned at Area A physical level alone and bundled the patient plus wife off with a prescription, but this would have indicated an excessively basic level of work which belies the depth of training a doctor should have had. Even a nurse or aide in under-doctored areas who has been taught "to treat all acute sore throats plus acute adenitis with penicillin" should be able to appreciate the value of extending the consultation into the other dimensions mentioned. When this happens, the "cookery-book approach to PHC" (see page 43) becomes replaced by a greater degree of professionalism and the principles of PHC begin to throw new light on difficult issues.

The reader will notice that in the case of John P., several dimensions were omitted from the consultation. The doctor made no attempt to deal in Areas C or D and even Area B was only invoked at the most basic level — that of trying to understand the factors and concerns which brought the patient to the doctor, what some authors call "ecognosis" (Stewart et al. 1975). The reasons for this were quite simple: that John P. had no continuing clinical problem (Area C) and attention to preventive care (Area D) would be inappropriate while the couple's attention was focused on a serious problem, the testicular lump; furthermore, their decisions about when to seek medical help were entirely appropriate (Area B). The patient's concern to interpret his symptoms in causal terms — "It was due to overwork doctor" — is indicative of how unsatisfactory a diagnosis of "streptococcal adenitis" can be to an intelligent patient who asks *why* this should occur (Balint 1964; Locker 1981). For the doctor, this was a pointer to the possibility that John P. had been feeling stressed or off-colour for longer than he had indicated.

Example 2: Strengthening Mothering

Example 2 illustrates very different aspects of the application of understanding medical help seeking (Area B). The setting is a township in south-east Africa, but it could have been chosen from elsewhere in the world.

Lisa (2 years) is brought to a clinic nurse by her mother because she is apathetic and having diarrhoea. The nurse realises that the child is suffering from protein–calorie malnutrition (PCM) as indicated by her weight, pitting oedema of the ankles, pigmentary skin changes and gingering of the hair. The infant has been treated by a local herbalist without success and is fourth in a family of five children, the youngest now being 8 weeks old.

The child's physical problems can be treated with appropriate food and the infective complications which often accompany PCM can also be cured by modern medical techniques. But is this the best approach?

In terms of the evidence from advanced PHC, it is usually inappropriate to use food supplements, special feeds, drips and intensive nursing, which often typify traditional treatment, because these wrench control from the child's mother and mystify a process which is really due to nutritional problems. Pioneers of alternative approaches point to the need to use the child's illness to help her mother discover simple nutritional truths (Stott 1959): that the child will usually get better with appropriate food alone. It is essential for a mother to discover that she holds the key to family health provided she is able to overcome cultural or environmental barriers to implementing the new ideas. To bring an ill child back to health with food and maternal care alone is a golden opportunity. Here the skills and attitudes of Areas B and D can conflict with conventional curative practices because the quickest and safest cure may increase the risks of recurrence, whereas slightly slower methods which strengthen the mother's role and change the professional role to "helper" rather than "healer" are more likely to produce long-term community health. A detailed review of the evidence for this principle will be found in Chapters 4 and 5.

Example 3: Continuing Care

Continuing care of chronic problems is a major weakness in many PHC services. The Royal College of General Practitioners, the American Academy of Family Physicians and equivalent bodies in other· countries have paid lip-service to the importance of continuing care but a glance at the records in many practices or PHC clinics will reveal that episodic medicine is still rife. The gap between the theory and practice of continuing care is probably widening as personal doctoring becomes more difficult to sustain in many parts of the world. However, even personal knowledge of patients does not guarantee good continuing care because the number of patients can be too great, or patient mobility can erode the clinician's efforts to know his patients, and doctors themselves often know less about their patients than they would admit, particuarly if records are very brief or nonexistent.

The only solution to this problem is wider acceptance of the importance of asking at every consultation: "Are there any continuing problems which I should be dealing with while the patient is here?". Patients often see the PHC services sufficiently frequently for this disciplined approach to ensure that a high proportion of chronic conditions is reviewed informally and without special clinics or follow-up appointments, especially if good clinical records are kept.

Mr Jones (40 years) was known to have a blood pressure in the "grey area" between normality and unequivocal hypertension but he had avoided all health services as much as possible and was reluctant to follow advice to attend for occasional blood-pressure checks. At his first consultation for 3 years (for a lacerated finger) he was treated by a nurse with sutures and a booster of tetanus toxoid. In most clinics that would have been all, but awareness of Area C and a clinical record which contained the past history, led to a diagnosis of hypertension (210/130) and referral to a doctor.

This action by the nurse could be very important for Mr Jones' health and longevity, provided he is prepared to receive appropriate regular treatment. He did not request or expect the blood-pressure review; a cut finger was his complaint, but the nurse used her skills and knowledge to widen the scope of the consultation to his great advantage in an era of relatively safe hypertension therapy.

A significant proportion of patients attending for PHC have continuing care needs which they do not mention (30%–40% in British general practice). Routine Area C practice is a discipline which will vary in sophistication with the training of the staff involved and with the organisation of the services (see Chap. 3), but every aide, nurse and doctor who has front-line responsibilities should be able to broaden consultations in this way. The traditional episodic care (Area A alone) of many clinics will then begin to change towards the broader functions of modern PHC which uses many contacts to review chronic and continuing problems.

Example 4: Integrating Care

A final example will be drawn from a general practitioner's surgery where Simon (4 years) is seen with a cough of two days' duration but is otherwise well and no signs are present in his respiratory system. Many doctors and nurses would prescribe some linctus or other mixture and send him on his way, but this would be inappropriate, for the following reasons.

1) Why did his mother bring Simon with this minor problem? If she really came for a cough mixture alone, she should be encouraged to use her own resources rather than depend on the doctor for such things — a menthol lozenge, a spoon of honey, or a drink of sweetened lemon, even a cup of water is often as effective as most proprietary cough mixtures. However, the public expectation for a magic bottle (Webb 1978) is a difficult problem and this is only likely to be changed by techniques which involve demystification of some medical practices and a greater emphasis on the body's natural defences and processes rather than cures (see Chap. 4). It is also possible that Simon's mother simply looked for reassurance that the illness was self-limiting, and there is good evidence that doctors overestimate patients' expectations for treatment and underestimate their need for information (see Chaps. 2 and 4).

2) A 4-year-old child needs to be looked at with the eyes of a clinical surveyor. Is his size compatible with norms? Does his relationship with his mother seem normal? Are his vision, hearing and activity normal? Has he had appropriate immunisation? Does he have a mouth with decay in it?

These are not technical or sophisticated questions, they can be answered by the alert clinician in seconds while answering the child's presenting problem, and reference to charts, tables, measurements or specialists is only necessary where there is reasonable room for doubt. This "Area D-type" of activity for a child of pre-school age can be achieved quickly and with reasonable accuracy by those who discipline themselves to consider the same issues in most 4 year olds seen. The eye and ear of experience then quickly identify the definite deviations from normal for more detailed assessment (see Chap. 5).

3) Simon's clinical notes show that he had one incompletely descended testicle, identified 2 years previously. This continuing problem merits a review which will only happen if the clinician is alert enough to be looking for indications for continuing care in the record (Area C).

The organisation of PHC services will have a powerful influence on the degree to which the framework can be used as an aide-memoire because this broad approach to the consultation introduces a need for skills and facilities which no one person will be able to execute. The doctor/nurse of first contact will have to be backed up by others who provide reinforcement of the practical or educational activities which are initiated in the consultation. Sometimes therapy will need to be administered, immunisations will have to be given, opportunities for lessons in child care and food preparation and special tests or counselling are all often conducted by members of the PHC team other than the front-line clinician who directs patients to team members. Even home gardening, sanitation, fencing, water conservation and recreational activities can become logical extensions of the consultation if patients have barriers to health which could involve modifications to these activities.

Community experiments which have shown the efficacy of demystification in medicine and its integration into the community have been conducted in the United Kingdom and in the less developed world — evidence which will be illustrated in Chapter 5. The projects which will be presented have in common: team-work, an educational emphasis, an attempt to evaluate the work, and the use of the consultation as a medium for motivation.

The four examples chosen for this chapter have been used to illustrate the principles of working beyond the presenting problem(s) (Area A), so every consultation can embrace other relevant disorders (Area C) and stimulate preventive activity in terms of care through appropriate help seeking (Area B) and screening or life-style changes (Area D). The framework is an aide-memoire to reinforce the potential in every consultation and clinicians who use it should take more opportunities for stimulating health awareness in the populations served. The theoretical and practical background to these four principles will be dealt with in the chapters which follow. It must, however, be emphasised that doctors alone cannot achieve more than part of the potential in every consultation. The clinician (whether nurse, nurse-practitioner or doctor) is the initiator and motivator but other tools, techniques and staff members have to facilitate what happens next. The degree of success will depend on the organisation and skills of the PHC team and the willingness of specialist units to provide back-up and moral support when the demands which are placed on those in PHC become so onerous that some PHC pressures have to be shifted on to secondary (specialist) care services. When this happens, the wise specialist or administrator will ask, not for more specialised resources, but for those things which strengthen PHC and "the family in society".

References

Balint M (1964) The doctor, his patient and the illness, 2nd edn. Pitman Medical, London
Bowling A (1981) Delegation in geneal practice. Tavistock, London
Department of Health and Social Security (1971) The organisation of group practice. Chairman R Harvard Davis. HMSO, London
Leeuwenhorst Working Party (1977) The work of the general practitioner. Statement by a working party appointed by the Second European Conference on the Teaching of General Practice. J Roy Coll Gen Pract 27:117
Locker D (1981) Symptoms and illness: the cognitive organisation of disorder. Tavistock, London
Royal College of General Practitioners (1972) The future general practitioner — learning and teaching. British Medical Journal, London
Stewart MA, McWhinney IR, Buck CW (1975) How illness presents. A study of patient behaviour. J Fam Pract 2(6):411
Stott HH (1959) A pilot health study of the Zulu community. Report to the Expert Committee on Public Health Administration. PHA/33. WHO, Geneva
Stott NCH, Davis RH (1979) The exceptional potential in each primary care consultation. J Roy Coll Gen Pract 29:201–205
Taylor R (ed) (1978) Family medicine. Springer-Verlag, New York
The General Practitioner in Europe (1974) Second European Conference on the Teaching of General Practice. Leeuwenhorst, Netherlands
Webb P (1978) Man, magic and the modern placebo. Health Educ J 37:165–168

3. From Episodic to Continuing Care

Introduction

"Continuing care" is the term applied to the care of patients with chronic problems and/or the management of acute illness which needs review on one or more occasions. Continuing care is, therefore, the antithesis of episodic acute medicine, and the need for continuing PHC increases as the number of people with chronic or disabling problems increases in the population. The term must not be confused with continuity of care which refers to the patient seeing the same doctor (or nurse or aide) in personal PHC or family medicine. Continuity of care does *not* guarantee good continuing care as many "personal PHC clinicians" have not adopted the skills, tools or discipline of continuing care. Unfortunately, the very nature of PHC tempts the clinician to allow his care to become episodic because so many patients come for help with one acute problem, and pressure of time can easily become a barrier or an excuse to avoid wider continuing care responsibilities in a high proportion of patients. Videotape recordings in British general practice have shown that only about one patient in seven has more than one problem handled at each consultation, and an analysis of medical records has shown how fewer than 50% of elderly patients have two or more problems considered when they attend for PHC, despite the chronic and recurring nature of their disabilities (Stott 1980).

Medical education is still geared primarily to the management of acute illness, leaving mental or physical handicap, personality disorders, degenerative diseases, psychosocial symptoms and terminal care to the fringes of medicine. Furthermore, the size of the pool of chronic disease in the community and the pressure of work often make PHC doctors reluctant to widen the content of their consultations to embrace problems which the patient is not actively complaining about. However, the expanding horizons of medicine have provided for the control of more and more conditions which need treatment for years or which merit periodic review to avoid complications. Prescribing patterns have also led to a generation of pill takers in many countries who are at special risk from the therapy they expect or depend upon, and the ageing populations of some countries need more and more symptomatic therapy to help them to weather the degenerative processes of old age and the stresses of industrialised society (Kohn and White 1976; Jones et al. 1980).

The PHC clinician who can turn his back on this tide of chronic human problems which require continuing supervision and who clings to an era of crisis intervention for acute problems is trying to hold PHC back from skills, tools and behaviours which are needed in the twentieth century, which enhance the rǫle of the discipline, and which separate it from the more limited disease-specific objectives of the specialties.

How can continuing care be encouraged?

1) By applying a professional discipline to every consultation.
2) By use of methods which facilitate continuing care.
3) By appropriate personal care and interpersonal skills (see Chap. 1).

These will be considered and their advantages and disadvantages discussed with illustrative examples from different cultures.

Continuing Care as Part of the Discipline of PHC

The most basic and simple way to achieve effective continuing care is when the clinician in PHC disciplines himself to consider whether there is a need for continuing care at every consultation. Without this discipline, the practice of continuing care has to depend on the patient requesting it or occur in an ad hoc fashion, practised only when there is time and inclination. The self-imposed discipline of the framework of the PHC consultation helps young clinicians to avoid the trap of episodic medicine (see Fig. 2.1).

In a nationalised health service where over two-thirds of the patients on a general practitioner's list are seen by him at least once every year, the opportunities for unobtrusive attention to continuing problems are enormous, and this is dealt with in more detail later. Even in a less organised and structured system, it is commonplace for PHC doctors, nurses or aides to have sufficient contacts with their patients to attempt similar objectives for a fair proportion of people seen, and without excessive duplication of effort as few patients attend several PHC physicians simultaneously and specialists will usually confine their continuing care to a single system.

A 3-year-old child with a past history of strabismus is seen by her family doctor with earache. She has only been seen once in the past 18 months for some minor ailment. The doctor may deal with the earache alone (Area A) or take the opportunity to review or arrange to review the child's vision, even though her mother had not come with this in mind (Area C). Both problems could be of great importance to the child's future development and to treat one without checking the other would seem strange practice.

Mary (32 years) had severe pre-eclamptic toxaemia (PET) with her first two pregnancies but now, 5 years later, comes to see her doctor about an attack of acute dysuria which is confirmed to be cystitis. The consultation moves beyond Area A if Mary's blood pressure is checked because with a history of PET she is still at risk for hypertension (Area C). In many clinics the cystitis would be treated in isolation and no consideration given to her being at continuing risk for other problems.

Even the most informed patients may underestimate the need for periodic review of chronic or relapsing problems, and so it is incumbent on every PHC clinician to use each patient contact for continuing care when this is appropriate because the practice is a highly efficient use of the consultation if viewed in terms of outcome for the patient. It also provides a constant source of clinical challenge to the doctor or nurse involved by widening the potential in every consultation.

When students are taught to consider the need for continuing PHC at every consultation as rigorously as the surgeon applies aseptic techniques in the operating theatre, they begin to identify three important phenomena which are necessary if professional standards are to be achieved.

1) That the practice of continuing care is inappropriate in certain situations.
2) That personal knowledge of the patient can help or hinder the practice of continuing care.
3) That continuing care depends in part on the availability of devices and methods which facilitate its practice (see p. 25).

It is, for example, inappropriate to practise continuing care when the problem the patient comes with is so severe or emotionally painful that attention to other less acute issues would seem to be an impertinence or an irrelevance.

John S. (42 years) has been killed in a car accident. His wife has consulted twice since the event and on each occasion you decide to deal with the acute grief only, ignoring the opportunities for continuing care of her recent menorrhagia which she seems to have forgotten about.

Peter F. (4 years) has been an erratic attender at clinic following severe malnutrition and he had persisting growth retardation when last seen 2 years ago. His family, who live in the mountains 6 miles away, bring him to you with an asthmatic attack.

In both these situations the correct medical approach is to attend to the crisis in hand and any thought of the continuing care of menorrhagia in Mrs S. or the developmental assessment of Peter F. has to be shelved until a more appropriate moment. However, most PHC is not crisis medicine and so this type of care is the exception rather than the rule. Most patients, once prompted, are very willing to accept review of problems beyond the immediate felt needs.

Personal knowledge of patients (continuity of care) should help to provide quick and relevant continuing care because, in theory, the clinician remembers the patient's history well and does not even need medical records to remember the problems (McWhinney 1978). Unfortunately, the evidence for this belief is shaky: doctors see too many people to remember details for long and they are much better at remembering recent acute events than the more chronic problems. Patients seen and remembered least may have continuing problems which are most in need of review: for example, in a study of 299 chronically ill patients, Stewart et al. (1979) were able to show that the doctors' knowledge of patients was best in those with a small number of problems, a large number of recent visits and a patient-initiated consultation. Continuity of care (personal care) is highly prized by many patients and a good case has been made by Perreira Gray (1979) for PHC doctors to have personal lists to enhance the quality of care. One assumption in Gray's approach is that personal care (continuity) is closely correlated with high-quality continuing care. In the articulate middle classes, this may sometimes be true, but it is much less likely to occur in the lower social groups who are less able or willing to help the doctor/nurse widen the PHC consultation to embrace more than the presenting problem (Pendleton and Bochner 1980). Indeed, it is also not uncommon for doctors to feel resentful about those patients who structure their consultations to embrace a series of unrelated problems.

Mrs Jones came in today with her shopping list of complaints and requirements . . . even a 15-minute appointment is insufficient to keep up with her multiple groans.

Excellence is undoubtedly the attractive combination of personal continuity of care with skilled continuing care, but sadly there is little evidence that the two are associated in more than a minority of PHC groups. The reasons for this are complex because changing social pressures and higher population mobility have reduced both the opportunities and the desire for creating a highly personal PHC in many areas. Sad though this change may be, it is a reality, and the skills of continuing care will still have to be learned by those who work in all types of clinical PHC, personal or less personal, urban or rural, affluent or poor. Each will have its special problems but the skills and methods which are necessary for continuing care will be similar in each case.

Familiarity and Familiarity Blindness

The advantages to the patient of continuity of care are difficult to prove, except by an audit of chronic-disease management and on the basis of patient satisfaction, but continuity must always be differentiated from familiarity. This is highlighted by the familiar anecdote of a student who was first to diagnose hypothyroidism in a patient who had seen the professor of medicine regularly for several years. We are often most blind to the needs of those nearest to us, and this great risk in clinical PHC can only be overcome by diligent refusal to become "stale" and by appropriate use of records which will prompt reconsideration of continuing problems which would otherwise be displaced by the more attractive, but often less important, acute illnesses or by irritation about very demanding patients. Perhaps the most important physical sign of dangerous familiarity is when the clinician's heart sinks as the patient enters — "heart-sink patients" are at risk for incomplete care because the clinician is often less alert when dealing with them by virtue of negative feelings.

Mrs S.P. (52 years) had been a regular attender and moaner at her family doctor's surgery for 20 years. Her records were fat with clinical notes and multiple specialist referrals — referrals which had exposed her to numerous procedures and operations and left her with abdominal ahesions and scars but without relief from her recurrent abdominal pain. When she started to tell her doctor yet again about her bowel problems, his heart sank and he paid little attention to her familiar groans and prescribed symptomatic therapy until her newly developing rectal carcinoma could almost be diagnosed without a proctoscope.

The PHC or family doctor who takes responsibility for continuing care of patients like Mrs S.P. has to use appropriate specialists and yet try to continue to provide care when others have failed and cure seems elusive or impossible. The trap of familiarity blindness in an evolving human situation is as unpleasant as any other diagnostic error, but its impact is accentuated by the prolonged agony of caring for the patient and family both before and after the doctor's failure to recognise that expertise can be diminished in quality by negative "heart-sink" attitudes. Some authors have labelled such patients "hateful patients" because their relationship with the health care providers is clinging, manipulating, rejecting and/or demanding (Groves 1978). Such words all reflect negative feelings in the primary health care provider and accentuate the need for clinicians to hold and to teach a clear policy for the recognition and management of such patients.

A study of the doctor–patient relationship and the complex transactions, bonds, tricks, power struggles and games which can be manifest in PHC doctoring is essential for any clinician who is striving to develop some understanding of the power and hazards of continuing care and continuity of care. Browne and Freeling's (1967) introduction to the subject is an outstanding primer to these principles, but many texts now deal with the same issues in other ways and a common thread which runs through such analyses is the need for the clinician to be secure enough to involve himself constructively in the patient's feelings. Some physicians find that this seems risky because it threatens their sense of control, and yet with training and experience these fears can be overcome and psychotherapeutic situations can be created where previously they were avoided.

To reach out to another person in emotional distress is to provide a life-line which helps him to work his way back to a less hazardous place. The life-line of sympathy can, however, become a tangled web of misplaced affection and fear if both clinician and patient do not accept that the life-line has to be reeled in and put away once the patient is standing safely on the shore of life once more. Continuing care of chronic and recurring problems, however, is an essential part of PHC which runs a constant risk of encouraging undue dependence on the doctor/nurse, but a plan which involves patients fully in their own care is less likely to create unhealthy dependency. Perhaps the most important lesson for PHC workers is that dependent and "heart-sink" patients are often difficult to understand when the clinician stands alone; sharing the problem with supportive colleagues and/or other health professionals will often help to begin to clarify a logical approach to the continuing problem. Sharing the difficulties with the patient openly will also sometimes precipitate remarkable results and pre-empt a disaster of misunderstanding about roles and expectations.

Methods Which Can Facilitate Continuing Care (Area C)

1) Recording methods.
2) Organisational methods.

1) Recording Methods

Reliable knowledge of patients' continuing problems can only come from a well-structured and orderly clinical record which is sufficiently concise and legible to ensure that continuing problems the patient fails to mention are not overlooked. The commonest barriers to achieving this method of communication are as follows.

1) A lack of agreed structure in medical records: clinicians treasure differences.
2) Fragmented PHC systems involving several health care providers.
3) Extremes of information gathering: either pitifully inadequate notes or volumes of excessive recording which smother essential clinical features.
4) Refusal to let the patient carry his/her own clinical record despite poorly co-ordinated care.
5) A belief that computers will solve the problem so any effort today will be wasted tomorrow.

Fortunately, most continuing care demands minimal recorded information and those who have tried to organise their records learn that many systems are unnecessarily complex. A place for a summary problem list which includes all episodes of ill-health of continuing relevance and a place for continuation notes to highlight the nature of each new problem are all that is required to achieve basic continuing care in most PHC clinics and practices, particularly if the decision to improve the medical record stimulates the PHC providers to discuss their objectives and agree to an outline record structure.

Perhaps the most disruptive element to co-ordinated continuing care is the trend in developed countries for more and more agencies or specialists to be involved with individual patients. This brings the merit of specialised skills and knowledge but the danger of duplication and inco-ordination which can reach a crisis point very quickly when patients are inarticulate or handicapped and thus unable to orchestrate their own health care. Shared-care records, which are kept in the patient's home or by relatives who have to deal with various professionals, are one simple solution to this fragmented care problem; each doctor, nurse or aide making simple entries on the common patient-held record. Antenatal shared-care cards are a well-tried example of this practice (Fig. 3.1), and hypertension flow charts are another (Fig. 3.2). Even complex

| | | Height .... Blood Group ...   Special points ....   Foetal Movements Felt............ |
| | | WR/KAHN/PPR .... Rhesus .... Bacilluria.............................. |

| | Weight | | | | | | | | | | | Next Visit (Weeks) | | |
Urine	lbs	kg	B.P.	Oedema	Maturity Weeks	Fundal Height	Presentation and Position	FH	Hb gms %	Remarks	GP	HSP	Initials

Fig. 3.1.   A patient-held monitoring card for antenatal care.

26

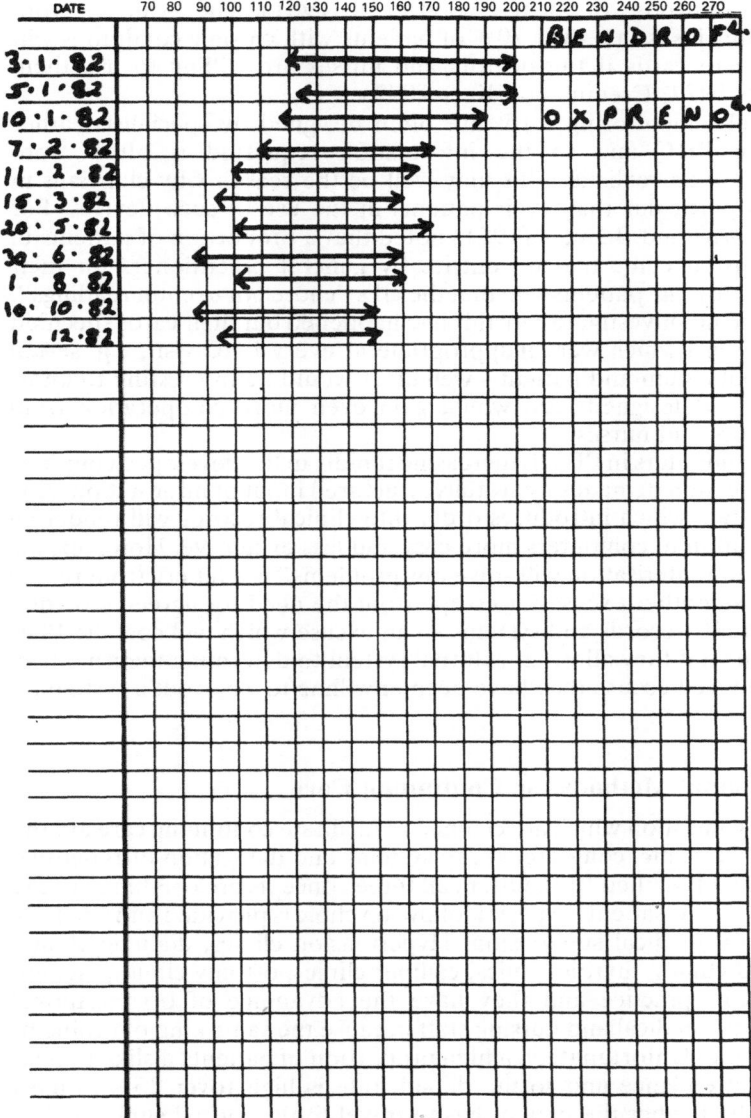

Fig. 3.2. A patient-held monitoring card for hypertension.

degenerative diseases lend themselves to this method if "clinic cards" are held by the patient. Does the card get lost? Occasionally, yes, but those who allege that patients are unreliable are usually suprised to find that it is the doctors rather than the patients who fail to use the continuing care record card consistently. Even illiterate tribal mothers can prove remarkably reliable in the use of self-held records about their children's growth and development if they

27

understand the purpose of them (Wood et al. 1981). The evidence from developed countries is that over 70% of patients with chronic conditions will carry shared-care cards if the doctors and nurses are willing to use them (Downie et al. 1977; Ezedum and Kerr 1977).

Unfortunately, monitoring cards are often designed by specialists rather than those in PHC and so the information requested is often more comprehensive than realistic. This may well be the reason why clinicians in PHC are less particular than their patients in the use of such devices. For example, Osborne and Beevers (1981) noted that a proportion of patients in their hypertension clinic had no entries by general practitioners on their shared-care cards. The patients said that the GPs "chose not to enter readings". The authors did not investigate *why* this had happened but their cards specified a number of items which were inappropriate at every PHC visit, e.g. serum urea, serum potassium and patient's weight. It would be interesting to know whether a better designed card would gain even more co-operation from patients, doctors and nurses.

The use of computers in PHC is increasing rapidly in the developed countries and each application demands a carefully structured input of information. Any traditional system which introduces order into clinical records will render an eventual transition to computers more easy and less expensive. However, the philosophy "computerisation will solve our problems" is a far cry from reality and represents another excuse for escape from the need for agreed structure and order in PHC records and systems — an excuse which will cost the PHC team a great deal if they allow an external system to determine their mode of work in the future because they have been unwilling to work out a system for themselves.

2) Organisational Methods for Continuing Care

Methods of organisation which are claimed to facilitate continuing care are the special follow-up clinic, computer recall systems and delegation of repetitive duties to less highly skilled staff. Often, all three concepts are combined as the computer recalls the patient, a special follow-up clinic is provided and ancillary staff run it with medical supervision. Hypertension clinics, diabetic clinics, developmental clinics, thyroid clinics, calliper clinics, ostomy clinics, etc. are examples of this practice and they have the advantage of organisational simplicity for the medical and nursing staff because the same kind of problems come to each one. Unfortunately, a high proportion of patients dislike regular special clinic attendance and so the default rate is high (over 25% in most centres) and the further the patient has to travel to the special clinic the less satisfactory the attendance pattern becomes (Gruer 1972). When special clinics form part of the local PHC service, the problem of access may be alleviated but the duplication of visits is not avoided as many patients have found that they have to attend on separate clinic days for different functions: Monday for immunisations, Tuesday for family planning, Wednesday for antenatal, Thursday for hypertension/diabetes, and Friday for developmental problems in children — quite daunting for the mother with a family of young children because the combination of fragmented preventive and continuing care is often most difficult for young mothers with problems (Fig. 3.3).

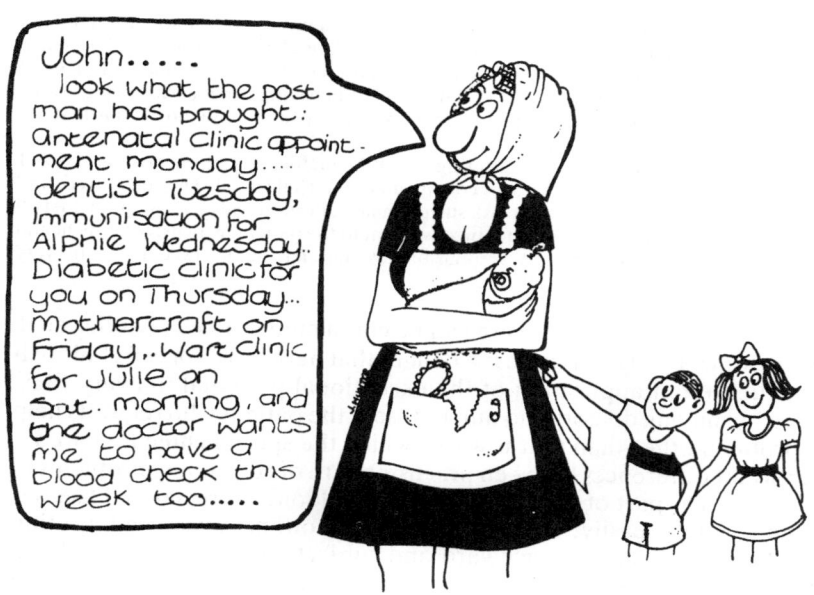

Fig. 3.3.

Specialised follow-up clinics have enjoyed a vogue in both developed and less developed countries because it is possible to train relatively unskilled staff to undertake major portions of the repetitive work which is generated. Compliance and attendance rates have sometimes shown that the patients find these clinics unsatisfactory for reasons that are complex but certainly include a lack of flexibility when patients want to consult about other problems, and the duplication of travel and waiting for those whose illnesses or family needs bring them to more than one clinic.

Primary health care in developed countries has adopted the special clinic approach on a wider scale than ever before, aided and abetted by the Royal College of General Practitioners and the postgraduate training schemes for PHC which have often regarded special clinics as a sign of progress. The fragmenting effect this may have on family care does not need to be spelt out further, but clearly a balance does need to be struck between the essential special clinic which provides a procedure for healthy people (for example immunisation) and the less successful special clinics (for example hypertension, epileptic, diabetic, thyroid, nutrition) where patients often need quite a broad and integrated approach to more complex problems, and so they need to be seen by people with a broad professional training who are not limited to one set of special skills or procedures.

Patients who default from follow-up from special clinics are often condemned as indolent or irresponsible, yet too often follow-up systems provide patients with long travel and waiting times, only to be seen by juniors or aides.

John P. (38 years), a well-controlled epileptic with a 5-mile journey to hospital, came in one morning after a long wait in an epilepsy clinic waiting room. A brief history was taken by a nurse who then took blood for a routine check. A young doctor entered next, nodded and said "This all looks fine . . . can we see you in 6 months?". John P. said "I'm having trouble with an ingrowing toe-nail", to which the young doctor replied, "You must see your own doctor about that".

After John P. had left, disgruntled and muttering about the inefficiency of the health service, I asked the young doctor why the patient was coming up to the clinic at all. The reply I received reflected amazement that I should need to ask such an inane question and an assumption that all epileptics need specialist care . . . even if it is inconvenient to the patient, expensive to the health service, errosive on the PHC team's responsibilities and having to take place in very overcrowded clinics with a high default rate.

Highly effective epilepsy after-care can be conducted in PHC (Zander et al. 1979; Lloyd-Jones 1980), yet there is a danger that here too a special clinic will grow and squeeze out application of the exceptional potential in every PHC consultation by making doctors and nurses resent the patient who requests help for some problem other than that towards which the special clinic is geared.

The important differences between practising care of continuing problems in special clinics and as part of generalist PHC are seldom appreciated. Diseases fit into clinics quite easily: routine questions, routine tests, and routine treatment. People are varied, awkward and subject to multiple interrelated problems which cannot be broken up into their component parts without risk of serious fragmentation and duplication: a minority of people do need the skills of the specialist but most need care which is accessible, acceptable and able to deal with more than one problem at a time (Fig. 3.4; Marson et al. 1973; Pritchard 1978).

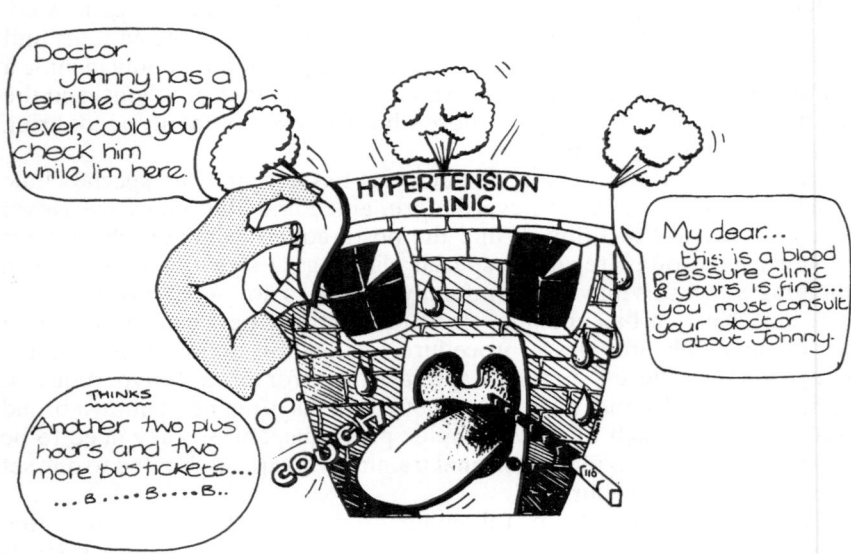

Fig. 3.4.

30

Can computers do more for continuing care than to generate reminders for patients who fail to attend for follow-up? The answer to this question is yes, because any device which can help the doctor/nurse/aide in PHC remember to deal with more than the presenting problem will increase the efficiency and effectiveness of each consultation. Unfortunately, computers are more often used in a way which generates additional appointments and contacts with PHC than to increase the power of existing consultations because of technological and practical limitations on their use as clinical records. Experiments which place all PHC clinical data on computer are still experimental and expensive, but it is possible that this will change with the advance of microtechnology. More difficult to change will be clinicians' willingness to accept disciplined continuing care imposed by computer programming!

Conclusions

Tools, methods and skills which help the doctor to conduct effective continuing care will obviously enhance professional judgement and performance, particularly when the doctor feels stressed by limited time. In this chapter, the advantages and disadvantages of the various strategies have been discussed but they can only operate optimally when applied together by a well-trained practitioner in a well-organised situation.

There is a danger that continuing care in the future may be left to the computer and/or the special clinic recall system instead of being based on professional vigilance and the kind of contractual arrangement between doctor and patient which ensures that both are aware of problems that need periodic review. Any system which helps the doctor identify patients who have greatly exceeded their review time will obviously be helpful, but it is inconceivable that review appointments can or should be sent out for more than a fraction of patients requiring review; first, because patients are not good at responding to recall for routine review; and secondly, because over the course of 3 years most PHC practitioners will see over 90% of their patients at least once, and every contact is an opportunity to deal with continuing problems. The doctor must ask himself whether there are continuing problems to be dealt with every time he sees his patient, and his records and staff should assist this professional discipline. Even where continuing care is delegated to aides or nurses, the same principles should apply because the primary plan of management will be made by the responsible clinician. Continuing care demands an awareness of the disciplines of primary medical care and the application of skills and methods which will improve the quality of the service offered. The application of Area C (see Fig. 2.1) is the first step from episodic medicine towards a more comprehensive approach to every consultation in the emerging discipline of PHC, and those forces in community and specialist medicine which encourage fragmentation of the consultation potential need to be resisted or modified.

References

Browne K, Freeling P (1967) The doctor–patient relationship. Churchill Livingstone, Edinburgh

Downie WW, Leatham PA, Rhind VM, Wright J (1977) Steroid cards: patient compliance. Br Med J 1:428–429

Ezedum S, Kerr DNS (1977) Collaborative care of hypertensives using a shared record. Br Med J 2:1402–1403

Gray PD (1979) The key to personal care. J Roy Coll Gen Pract 29:666–677

Groves JE (1978) Taking care of the hateful patient. New Engl J Med 298:883–887

Gruer R (1972) Outpatient services in the Scottish Border Counties. Scottish Health Service Studies, No. 23. Scottish Home and Health Department, Edinburgh

Jones DA, Sweetnam PM, Elwood PC (1980) Drug prescribing by general practitioners in Wales and in England. J Epidem Comm Health 34:119–123

Kohn RF, White KL (eds) (1976) Health care — an international study. Oxford University Press, London

Lloyd-Jones A (1980) Medical audit of the care of patients with epilepsy in one group practice. J Roy Coll Gen Pract 30:396–400

McWhinney IR (1978) Continuity of care in family practice. J Fam Pract 2(5):373

Marson WS, Morrell DC, Watkins CJ, Zander LI (1973) Measuring quality in general practice. J Roy Coll Gen Pract 23:23–31

Osborne VL, Beevers DG (1981) A comparison of hospital and general practice blood pressure reading using a shared-care record card. J Roy Coll Gen Pract 31:345–350

Pendleton D, Bochner S (1980) The communication of medical information in general practice consultations as a function of patients' social class. Soc Sci Med 14A:669–673

Pritchard P (1978) Manual of primary health care: its nature and organisation. Oxford University Press, London, pp 11–20

Stewart MA, McWhinney RI, Buck C (1979) Doctor–patient relationship and its effect on outcome. J Roy Coll Gen Pract 29:77–82

Stott NCH (1980) Clinical audit in two teaching health centres. Unpublished data

Wood CH, Vaughan JP, de Glanville H (1981) Community health. African Medical and Research Foundation, Nairobi

Zander LI, Graham H, Morrell DC, Fenwick P (1979) Audit of care of epileptics in general practice. Br Med J 2:1035–1039

4. Help Seeking: How, Where, Why, Wither?

The patient's decision to seek help is often made against a fairly complex background and yet those who are consulted can be surprisingly limited by their poor insight into the help-seeking process.

> "Patients come to see me because I'm the best doctor in town" said one flambuoyant colleague, to which one of his patients retorted under her breath "Only because you are most easily available."

In the less developed areas of the world where PHC is nonexistent or strictly limited, the ability to choose a service does not even exist and professional monopolies can be associated with a tragic lack of accountability unless there exists outstanding integrity in the person(s) concerned. Understanding help seeking will not assist in the acquisition of integrity but it will help the young doctor who is developing his ideas and skills to find the PHC task more fascinating and logical than would otherwise be possible: this chapter will be concerned with meanings, places and perspectives in help seeking.

The Meaning of Health and Illness

Perhaps the most ill-understood determinant of help seeking is the interpretation (meanings) the public attach to their symptoms and illnesses. Few Western clinicians even elicit such information at routine clinical interview: so powerful is the scientific biomedical concept of disease causation that any other interpretation of causation or meaning seems trivial, inappropriate or primitive. This attitude may be valid in organic terms but it provides nothing except a communication barrier if the patient holds beliefs or interpretations of health and illness which make traditional clinical recommendations look illogical or inappropriate. The attitude also traps medical thinking into a framework which is often intolerant of other approaches, a view which is neither scientific nor sensible because many of the most pressing health problems are concerned with choices and behaviour.

No attempt will be made to review the considerable literature on the questions people need answered about health and illness, but the relationship these have with help seeking in PHC and the contribution they may make to clinical work are our concern and so the following aspects will be considered.

33

1) The differences between illness, disease, sick role and health.
2) Traditional healers, self-care and PHC.
3) Explanations of health and illness.

1) Illness, Disease, Sick Role and Health

Sociological tradition now separates concepts of illness (the patient's subjective feelings of ill-health) from disease (the pathological processes defined in various clinical ways) and the sick role (a term used to denote inability to perform usual social functions due to ill-health). Western medical doctors are often accused of being interested in disease only, although the basis for such accusations is probably more orchestrated than justified because many PHC clinicians and other physicians are not bound by tight mechanistic biomedical ideas despite the benefits of biomedicine which have been sufficiently impressive to make its concepts fairly dominant. A crude illustration of the three terms used to describe ill health would be:

> Mrs Jones (23 years) is agitated by her recurrent dysuria and frequency which is very upsetting (the illness). Her doctor diagnoses a urinary infection due to *Esch. coli* (the disease) and advises 3 days off work because she works in an environment where she cannot get to the toilet easily (the sick role).

> Mr Peters (30 years) works as a labourer and has sprained his back. He feels unable to work but does not feel that a doctor will help. His wife is unsympathetic about him staying at home unless he consults a doctor, whereas he feels that a couple of restful days will do the trick: i.e. he wants to adopt the sick role for 2 days but his wife says no. (The definition or authorisation of sick role is not necessarily a medical matter!)

It is important for students to learn that the process of feeling ill, deciding to seek help, becoming labelled with a disease and being pronounced "off sick" is a sequence which most patients in PHC do not fulfil and moreover each phase can be independent of the others (Balint 1964; Wadsworth et al. 1971; Banks et al. 1975; Mechanic 1978; Journal of the Royal College of General Practitioners 1982).

a) Over two-thirds of people who feel ill do not seek help from professionals in most societies (Fig. 4.1).
b) Many of those who seek help from professionals come for reasons other than illness (e.g. housing, preventive procedures, certification, etc.).
c) Many people with diseases are asymptomatic and therefore unaware of their "illness' or unwilling to accept it.
d) Certification of sickness bears more relationship to expressed distress than to either illness or disease: it can be a form of social manipulation, a valid marker of disease or a manifestation of personal problems.

The practical importance of the terms illness, disease and sickness is still relatively small but they are widely used by academics and research workers so students need to be able to apply them in the context of PHC and understand the implications.

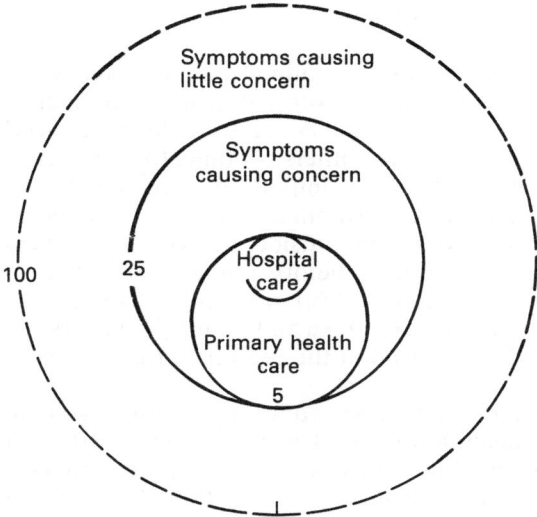

Fig. 4.1. Interfaces in health and illness. (Modified Horder and Horder 1954.)

Health is a very ambiguous concept because experience has shown that most people will talk about illness or the absence of illness when asked about "health". Pill and Stott (1982) found that mothers were much more confident when talking about their illness experiences than when asked about what they did to remain healthy. Nearly half of a sample of working-class mothers interviewed had no convincing views about personal choices which were exercised in the interests of health; they seemed to live within a very fatalistic framework accepting that ill-health was "bad luck" or "just one of those things", and that good health was a gift of fate rather than something to be worked for. The Social Class III Welsh mothers in this study had attitudes to health which were somewhat similar to those expressed by British university students when asked to relate how they would explain common illnesses to a child (Stacey 1978). In contrast, a similar study among American college students showed that they felt rather responsible for their health and resistance. A battle between the host defences and the "disease" was perceived by American students who seemed to fight for their health conceptually, whereas their British equivalents took it for granted. How much such differences are the product of cultural attitudes and how much they depend on education or social status is difficult to say, but wide variations do occur in the same cultural and social-class groups (Pill and Stott 1982) and the success of advertising certainly shows that people are prepared to be flexible in some choices they make. The relationship between help-seeking behaviour and a personal orientation to health is far from clear. It would be attractive to postulate that healthy minded and able-bodied people place fewer demands on the illness services, but the evidence for this assertion is incomplete and awaits confirmation in cross-cultural research.

2) Traditional Healers, Self-care and PHC

Whenever PHC is established it is superimposed on other traditional sources of advice or treatment of illness: stoicism, will-power, faith, home remedies, self-medication, fatalism, self-help, spiritual healers, advice/help from social networks, herbalists, acupuncturists, and many others continue to play a part, in even the most sophisticated of societies. It is important to realise that in every culture there is a variety of healers from whom a lay person can choose. Elliott-Binns (1973) estimated that advice from outside the Western medical service was taken from two to three sources before attending the British general practitioner. The proportion (about 75%) who use self-treatment before consulting is the same as that found in Mexican Indians (Young 1980) and other cultures (Kohn and White 1976), but the reasons for consulting a doctor may differ substantially.

Unfortunately, Western medicine is not renowned for its sensitive handling of relationships with traditional healing sources. Those who have worked in underdeveloped areas will be aware of how easy yet unnecessary it is to have poor relationships with traditional medicine men/women, although it has been shown that avoidance of criticism and a desire to work without undermining the prestige of traditional healers in the local community can produce remarkable results (Stott 1976):

> The Valley Trust sociomedical experiment among the Zulu introduced Western PHC with a strong nutrition–agricultural thrust to help combat rising malnutrition problems. A policy was established in 1950 to avoid criticism of or fraternisation with traditional healers. Ten to 15 years later some Zulu medicine men and women were promoting the nutrition education and food production policies which had been introduced by the Trust by instructing their patients and trainees in the same methods.

Traditional healers are highly individualist in most cultures — no two curers are alike according to some anthropologists — but they are important because they often influence the views patients have and sometimes in a very positive way:

> Mr P. was obviously most unhappy about the explanations offered by the Professor of Medicine about the mechanism of his migraine. "I don't understand why my arteries should go into spasm . . . it must be to do with my liver." The family doctor, hearing the comment, said "Your liver (?)" and Mr P. proceeded to explain his belief in toxic metabolites from the liver circulating around the body — a notion obtained from a local naturopath. This concept had coincided with Mr P.'s own beliefs and had become a major barrier to accepting symptomatic therapy from the Professor "unless it improved the excretion of the offensive toxic metabolites". Fortunately for Mr P., his intolerance of nuts was easily recognised when a diet and migraine diary were kept for 2 weeks. This fulfilled his need to eliminate something which could be seen to be "toxic" and also produced a much lower frequency of migraine attacks.

In this case, the "elimination" of something perceived as toxic was a necessary prerequisite to healing and, fortunately, the medical and lay concepts coincided and balance was restored in practical and conceptual terms.

Traditional healers and lay support networks are important modifiers of help seeking because advice is sometimes given about when to consult a Western doctor. Elliott-Binns (1973) and Helman (1978) have both presented evidence to show that, in the United Kingdom, there is a tendency for less dependence on lay support and more on PHC. This finding is compatible with trends in the national morbidity surveys (Crombie et al. 1975) and it is often used to show how PHC services are being expected to handle too many minor ailments. Also, young mothers may be using the pharmacist for advice rather than their own mothers (Blaxter and Paterson 1982). Education for self-care is being advocated by some clinicians and sociologists as an answer to this dilemma (Danaher 1979; Katz 1979) but illness behaviour has not yet been shown to be an either/or phenomenon. Patients will not always use either self-care or PHC, instead many of them can enjoy the educational benefits of self-care and use the PHC services as well:

Mrs P: Peter (5 years old) had a temperature last night doctor and I gave him fluids and aspirin as the book on self-care said. He is a bit better today but I thought that I would come to have him checked to see if he is all right.

This parent applied the advice of the self-care manual but lacked the confidence to believe that her child was really back on the road to health. The PHC services needed to provide something more — a reinforcement that she (the mother) was doing the right things and that most minor ailments do not need medical intervention in healthy children. Self-care, lay support, traditional healers and modern medicine are often used sequentially or simultaneously in all kinds of cultures (Elliott-Binns 1973).

In every culture there is a variety of healers to choose from and the lay public do not always classify this range of choices into markedly different styles. Blumhagen (1980) has shown that differences between Western medicine and traditional healing systems are often more theoretical than real if viewed from the lay public's perspective because such striking individualism occurs between individual clinicians. The professional freedom which makes this diversity possible leaves room for patients to negotiate their care and then turn to other healers if the first one fails to relieve their distress. Specialists are quite accustomed to this type of consumer trading if they or the patient feel that there is nothing more to offer. Those in PHC who have an image of themselves as the providers of primary and continuing care to a defined population are sometimes offended to find that their patients resort to more than one source of healing, but doctors can have quite unrealistic concepts of their dominance in society and expressions like "my patients" probably have more meaning to the doctor than to his clientele. How often do doctors speak of "my patients" while patients speak of "the doctor"? It is an honour indeed to be called "Dr Jones" or "Dr Margot" in urban practice.

" . . . His blood pressure may be fine doctor but his hypertension is terrible." (Angry wife whose husband had well-controlled high blood pressure but was far from pleasant to live with.)

In this example the doctor achieved good blood pressure control but he was not very understanding about tensions in the household and the couple subsequently found peace in a spiritual healing group: but the patient stopped hypertensive therapy and suffered a minor cerebrovascular accident before the doctor saw him again 2 years later. The public's use of a variety of healers is often desirable, but those who work in modern PHC have to be aware of the phenomenon of shopping around and anticipate the possible adverse results of people finding a nonmedical healer who is trusted more than the medical man or woman. Sometimes this is quite unavoidable, but an understanding attitude in the doctor to folk beliefs, traditional healers and curious concepts of disease may make it possible for patients to enjoy the best of all systems of care rather than the worst. Fears and prejudices can then be discussed rather than acted out.

The author knows a patient with endocrine and cardiovascular disease who attends the clinic of the Professor of Medicine, a naturopath and a homeopath, but uses the family doctor to help to decide whether any of the various therapies are likely to interact adversely.

The implications of this approach will be returned to later.

3) Explanations of Health and Illness

Considerable fluidity of thought and action seems to occur in the lay-mind when faced with illness or with a health-related decision and this differs substantially from the systematic biomedical approach to health problems.

The desire of scientists to classify illness beliefs by content is rather like trying to classify the fish in an aquarium by their position — there is constant movement which can only be understood within the overall context and by taking cognisance of pressures on the individuals. Personal decisions about choice of healer or explanation of cause often appear pragmatic or even contradictory because they may seem to defy the systematic thinking of biomedical logic; nevertheless, they usually confirm the ways of a given culture. Those in PHC who have a deep grasp of their subject should be able to understand these paradoxes (which are more apparent than real) and to accept that many of the words which are used in the consulting room or methods of management which have been passed on by more senior colleagues will not appear in textbooks until the medical profession stops pretending that it is above lay beliefs.

That's a nasty wet cough Mrs Jones . . . let me dry it up with a little treatment. (Dr A.)

Doctor I've got a terrible cold . . . my head is thick and my nose runs like a tap. Just wrap up warm and I'll give you something to help turn the tap off. (Dr B.)

These are not medical explanations, they are common responses in the folk idiom of minor ailments in Britain and many other countries. Common infective illnesses have, for generations and in many cultures, been perceived in terms of being "wet" or "dry", "hot" or "cold", and lay remedies have abounded which "wet the dry", "dry the wet", "cool the hot" and "warm the cold" — usually with home remedies (Cosminsky 1975; Helman 1978).

Closely allied to this have been ideas of blame and responsibility, the older generations regarding "colds" as due to carelessness in allowing exposure to the elements whereas "fevers" are due to contact with other people and carry no connotation of personal carelessness or responsibility (Helman 1978). The language of the doctors in the above two examples is in the folk idiom of "drying up the wet symptom" and "warming the chill or cold". This is not the language they were taught in medical school, but most PHC doctors have no difficulty in combining scientific theories of causation with the folk ideas of cold or chill which invades or upsets the body: they integrate two concepts to fit the patients' beliefs, ideas and language.

The marrying of scientific theories and folk concepts in the language of minor illness has been associated with two interesting phenomena which may be causally linked.

1) The displacement of some simple home remedies by pharmaceutical products.
2) Claims that modern medicine is influencing too many aspects of normal life.

An advertisement for two different pharmaceutical cough mixtures (Fig. 4.2) illustrates how commercial groups have been quick to adopt concepts of

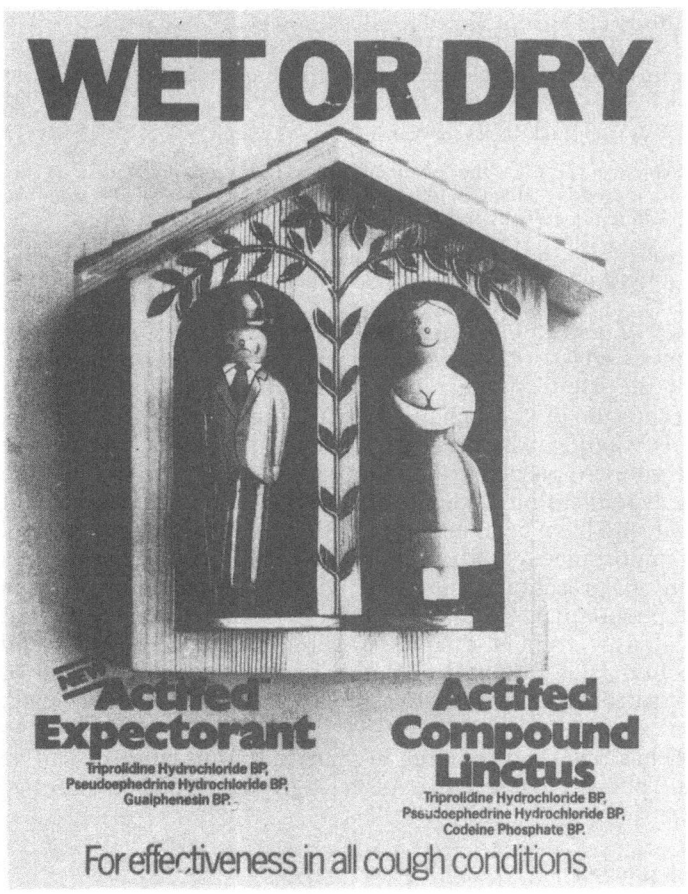

Fig. 4.2. "Wet or dry". A commercial application of a lay health belief.

"wet and dry" in folk idiom and thereby use the public's desire for medication. The fact that simple warm drinks, menthol, lemon and honey or other home-based ingredients, would usually do the same task at less cost and risk is important because a mother who depends on the pharmacy or doctor for such simple remedies has lost a fragment of her independence, resourcefulness and (perhaps) status. The ritual of preparing hot drinks or cold-packs or heating fruit juice cordials for an ailing child or relative is probably restoring to both mother and patient: in folk idiom she may be "flushing out" or "restoring balance" so the body can return to its previous healthy state. Helman (1978) has suggested that the modern symptomatic remedies from doctors or pharmacists are displacing some older healing traditions in Western societies and are encouraging modern medicine to invade and erode maternal confidence.

Salicylates will "sweat the illness out". Cough mixtures will "dilute or flush the illness'. Antidiarrhoeal mixtures will "dry it up".

Folk ideas and methods are not always harmless however:

The Zulu will "smoke" an ill child under a blanket to the point of intoxication and suffocation to drive out illness.

The Welsh will sometimes stop fluids in severe diarrhoea to "dry it up".

The hyperpyrexial techniques used in the treatment of malaria and pneumonia in the pre-antibiotic days were a crude resultant of folk ideas of "sweating it out" and a primitive medical approach to "killing the germ by heat".

Some African groups will pass a sharpened reed into the rectum of a child with constipation or dysentery and rotate it vigorously to release the internal "problem".

The consequences of medical involvement in lay-healing practices have therefore been double edged: it has commercialised and made medically dependent some of the useful home remedies and begun to modify some harmful rituals. Perhaps the greatest challenge which lies ahead for the young discipline of PHC is whether we can strengthen the lay public's roles and practices which are good — particularly in mothering — without making the population feel too dependent on medicine or commerce for the management of ailments which can and have been managed within the lay-healing network. The issue has great importance to both patients and PHC staff because there is evidence that incautious prescribing and poor job satisfaction among doctors are closely related phenomena (Melville 1980). It is likely, therefore, that unhappy or inadequately trained doctors undermine the confidence and traditional resourcefulness of patients by offering inappropriate treatments or by failing to provide satisfactory answers to essential questions about ill-health experiences.

Kleinman (1979) has reviewed research in many different cultures and he has shown that all people, irrespective of background, need answers to questions such as:

What caused this illness?
Why did it begin at a particular time?
What is happening to me?

What will be the outcome of this illness?
What should be done about it?

The individual searches to find answers to such questions and the explanations accepted by the individual will not be static. The explanatory ideas will change with remarkable rapidity as experiences change and the treatment options will vary accordingly. To the scientifically trained Western clinician who has never experienced serious illness himself, this switching and overlapping of hypotheses and treatments may seem irrational, but Kleinman points out that the sick individual seems to suffer no cognitive strain while holding so many options simultaneously. Furthermore, the first question is seldom satisfactorily answered in biological terms: pneumonia may be caused by an organism (= the mechanism or pathogenesis) but why was the organism able to invade at a particular moment? Why should this happen to me? Such questions delve into host/environment relationships and even into meta-physical and spiritual domains for some people, although lay folk are often reluctant to voice their fears.

In Taiwan, an individual will often use a traditional Chinese doctor, a religious Shaman and a Western physician at the same time.

In Scotland, a final-year medical student from Nigeria had Hodgkin's disease diagnosed and promptly departed for Ibadan to consult the family traditional healer. He returned later for conventional therapy and was much happier.

Mabry (1964), who conducted some of the classical work on lay concepts of illness causation, has, however, emphasised that apparent ignorance or evasiveness may be due to uncertainty rather than to a pure lack of knowledge; people may be well informed about the facts and hold two or more different interpretations of them but nevertheless appear to be ignorant because they are uncertain about which one is correct, particularly if the ideas threaten their beliefs and previous actions. For example, new dietary recommendations which contradict a previous pattern could imply that mother of the household has been incompetent unless great tact is exercised in helping her to modify her food choices and culinary skills. Mabry has also pointed to the heterogeneity of explanations about illness causation, showing that in his sample only 30% of husbands and wives could agree! Urban dwellers were more likely to attribute illness to environmental factors and factors under personal control than the rural dwellers who accepted "germs", "viruses" and "nerves" as common agents of illness. There are, however, powerful social and educational factors which modify health beliefs and which could explain some of Mabry's findings.

We see from this brief overview that two cardinal features of ill-health are (1) the search for restoration of balance, and (2) the pursuit of meaning in adversity.

Western medicine has not displaced the traditional beliefs and practices but it has begun to modify and even confuse many of them. It is pointed out later in this chapter that "germs" are still deeply misunderstood and ideas of medical power over them is often distorted as the popular image of a "virus" or "a bug" or "a germ" is of something that is susceptible to modern antibacterial therapy. Host resistance is underplayed in many biology lessons and consulting rooms, and the public is sometimes most resentful if a modern doctor does not exhibit

41

his therapeutic weapons when the illness is infective. Nevertheless, traditional ideas of "a balance of forces" being operative in both health and illness still lie deep in most cultures and disenchantment with modern medicine's magic bullets can be readily substituted by richer concepts which build on more complex ideas of how to restore balance in sick individuals, particularly the role of endogenous resistance rather than magic bullets (drug therapy).

The following are illustrations to show the duration and cultural diversity of the principle of balance.

The Chinese "Yin and Yang" represent the opposing forces of hot and cold, positive and negative, hard and soft, black and white, wet and dry, waxing and waning: in health each is seen to be in a state of balance and only when this is upset can pathogens invade. A concept which is 2500 years old!

The Greeks (Plato) held the belief that moderation in all things maintained a bodily balance and health. Therapy aimed to restore balance.

The Zulu live in balance with their ancestors and only if this is disturbed can an illness or ill-fortune supervene. Healers' rituals are aimed at the correction of imbalance, sometimes by placating angry ancestors.

In Yoga, complex exercises have been devised to restore muscle balance and to correct the inequalities of function which are often seen in the human body in the form of backache, stiffness, headaches, nervous tension, etc.

Many Latin Americans of Spanish origin believe that the healthy body is in an equilibrium state of hot and cold qualities, and foods are classified according to their hot/cold properties. Illness results from an excess of hot or cold in the body and cures are achieved by application of opposites.

The common thread of balance in health and imbalance in illness is so fundamental in many cultures that any attempt to modify ideas of causation, treatment practices or prevention should take serious cognisance of this deep-seated phenomenon. Simplistic ideas of single-factor causation have been a red herring to medical scientists and are also incompatible with many folk traditions and beliefs. It is indeed paradoxical that as medical scientists move towards more and more complex and multifactorial ideas of illness causation, so are they becoming more aware of the wisdom of the traditional systems which believe in balancing forces at work, and periods of susceptibility occurring when good balance is missing for some reason.

In concluding this section, it must be emphasised that the importance of health beliefs and folk practices does not lie in their classification. The deep-seated ideas of balance seem to be the only really universal generalisation; for the rest, ambiguity and fluidity are more characteristic features of lay persons' concepts of health and illness with a colourful overlay of culturally specific beliefs from which examples have been taken to illustrate various points. Life is an ambiguous affair — many daily situations are full of ambiguity and this becomes intolerable unless some meaning is applied to make sense of it (Locker 1981). The abundant theories of sick role, illness behaviour, labelling, attributions, stigma attachment, stress and health behaviour (to mention but a few) are a reflection of divergent research results and various schools of thought which are attempting to bring some scientific coherence to diverse ideas. The fact of ambiguity and the need to explain it in everyday life are, in this author's view, the most important findings because they help to make us understand the deep search for meaning that is part of individual lives, particularly in illness, ill-fortune and death. Ambiguity is also closely allied to "balance" because opposing forces can be in balance yet utterly ambiguous when considered from different viewpoints. Ambiguity is also compatible with complex multicausal concepts of causation which form part of many lay explanations and are increasingly espoused by medical scientists as they unravel the factors which underlie any one illness.

The professional in PHC cannot afford to look at problems from a purely biomedical viewpoint or he will be like the disciple who had eyes but would not see. The excitement, challenges and satisfactions in PHC appear when an understanding of the biomedical meets the "other half", the world of folk belief, searches for meaning and even spiritual experiences. The risk in this broad perspective is of being neither biomedical scientist nor traditional healer, a half-way house of bastardised disciplines. However, the alternative is to condone for ever the total separation of the two and to kindle professional blindness to the duality of man just as the young discipline of PHC is coming of age to recognise that it can draw the two together. The scientific validity of many sociological theories will find no better testing ground than the bench of PHC with its interfaces (Fig. 4.1), its ambiguous use of biomedicine and its traditions of pragmatic independence from rigid structuring.

What Is the Practical Importance of Having an Understanding of Help Seeking?

One of the objectives of the framework (see Fig. 2.1) is to highlight the fact that the experiences patients have in their consultations with a doctor or nurse may influence their expectations and their willingness to seek help in the future. The strength and the significance of consulting experiences will vary greatly from person to person and place to place, but many people attend for PHC in a worried and receptive frame of mind. The doctor/nurse who remains aware of this important phenomenon is using a most valuable asset because every management plan can provide either a conventional clinical solution or one that takes many longer term issues into account — issues which may influence the nature of PHC services and their efficacy because, as a front-line service, PHC can only function well if there is a balance between supply and demand which is rational and humane.

In recent years, medical practice has come under attack from philosophers (Illich 1977), industrial groups (Office of Home Economics 1975), the legal profession (Kennedy 1981) and from within the ranks of the profession (Crombie et al. 1975; Kohn and White 1976) for functioning in a way which encourages the dependence of the public on health care for trivial complaints. This medicalisation of many simple problems has been attributed to the philosophy of a "pill for every ill" or "medical redress for every distress" and those working in PHC have had much criticism levelled at them for practising in a cookery book way. Examples of cook-book practices are shown in Table 4.1, but it must also be said that anyone who has worked under the pressure of a

Table 4.1. Examples of the cook-book approach to symptom relief in acute "illness"

Distressing symptom	Relieving prescription
Coryza	Decongestant
Diarrhoea	Antidiarrhoeal
Constipation	Laxative
Pain	Analgesic
Wet cough	Expectorant
Dry cough	Cough suppressant
Unhappiness	Antidepressant
Anxiety	Anxiolytic
Malnutrition	Supplementary nutrients
Insomnia	Hypnotic

busy PHC clinic will realise that the ease of modern therapy coupled with patients' determined search for relief from distressing symptoms can place great pressure on the compassionate clinician to follow a symptomatic approach in the belief that it is caring medicine. The tragedy is that relief of symptoms can become a goal in itself and even smother the continuing need to ask why, how and how long? Furthermore, it is often unnecessary for a professional person to decide on therapy which is either unneccessary or which is available in the folk form or from the corner shop. Primary care personnel do, however, have a responsibility to encourage people to be more confident in their decisions and even in their home remedies especially when such confidence is lacking or shaken. Medical redress for every distress does not improve self-esteem or confidence in the recipient unless it helps the individual to understand more and to cope better.

Primary physicians are by no means the sole providers of excessive remedies as specialists are frequent users of therapies for so-called minor conditions which lie outside their specialty: steroid creams, cough mixtures, antidepressants, hypnotics, and β-blockers are common examples of prescriptions which are often recommended inappropriately. Perhaps the most pernicious example of all comes in tranquillisers which are frequently given to patients for no satisfactory reason. Balint (1964) commented on this phenomenon when he saw how angry some general practitioners became when a specialist, being unable to make a satisfactory diagnosis, proceeded to recommend some pseudopsychiatric treatment rather than admit inability to diagnose the problem. Balint wondered whether the specialists, being natural successors to the doctor's teachers, found it impossible to admit to inability to make a diagnosis.

The extensive use of medicines, prescribed and nonprescribed, is a world-wide problem which is well illustrated in a 12-nation survey by Kohn and White (1976). They demonstrated that in all countries, rich or poor, developed and less developed, a craving could be found for cures and potions to relieve distress: the most commonly sought were for cough and cold remedies, skin ointments and pain relief. A belief in the relief of distress by medicinal means is deep in most folklore and doctors often feel that patients are unrealistic in this belief. Nevertheless, studies into the prevalence of symptoms and illness in the general population reveal that only between 10% and 30% of clinical problems are brought to the PHC services, the rest being managed by ignoring them or by resorting to self-care, family advice, or other sources of lay information about health and illness (Fig. 4.1; White et al. 1961; Wadsworth et al. 1971; Hulka et al. 1972; Banks et al. 1975). Indeed, a shift of 10%–15% towards consulting with the professional PHC services would produce an overwhelming work crisis, hence the public's help-seeking behaviour is of more than academic interest!

Specialists and some pharmaceutical companies have become increasingly involved in this dangerous zone for many years; the former by conducting research on selected patients and then extrapolating their findings into the primary care sector, the latter by using the specialists' indiscretion. A recent notable example of this phenomenon is in the treatment of gastroenteritis with oral replacement therapy (ORT). For years, informed and experienced practitioners have advocated clear fluids with minimal sodium content for the vast majority of patients with acute diarrhoea and vomiting; various personal choices of mixture have been used but many have used ingredients which are available at home, often just clean water with flavouring and sometimes minimal added sugar and salt. Lack of precision in the preparation of these mixtures has occasionally led to the use of dangerously hypertonic solutions but the vast majority are grossly hypotonic and very suitable for prevention of dehydration in most diarrhoeal illnesses. Moreover, the mixing ritual of home ingredients keeps the power in "mother's" hands and helps her maintain self-esteem and the confidence of her family.

Paediatricians inevitably encounter more patients who have taken inappropriate antidiarrhoea drugs or antibiotics or who have been given hypertonic solutions. That this is the tip of a very small iceberg seems to have eluded the enthusiasts who have been advocating instead that "ideally every household should have a few packets of glucose–electrolyte powder . . ." and " . . . demands from parents for 'medicine' may be satisfied safely by prescribing a glucose–electrolyte mixture, such as X". Such generalisations in scientific journals have aided a vigorous pharmaceutical promotion campaign in the United Kingdom, and no doubt elsewhere too, to encourage the use of a commercial glucose–electrolyte solution in the *primary* treatment of diarrhoeal illness, particularly in general practice. The real population iceberg is the 70% of diarrhoea and vomiting which never comes near PHC and resolves spontaneously. To encourage a belief in prescriptive treatment rather than home fluids is to run the risk of repeating the errors of the past and to undermine further the common sense of many mothers and their grandmothers in the management of a condition which is rarely serious. Huge numbers of additional consultations for the provision of packets which are unnecessary for over 90% of the potential users may be a flattering goal for those specialists who promote such inappropriate dreams and it is good news for the commercial firms, retailers and wholesalers who market the products. However, such inadvertent collusion between specialists and commerce at the expense of PHC and of those mothers who need confidence reinforced in simple home remedies should be condemned. A similar phenomenon has occurred in relation to cough mixtures, tranquillisers, antipyretics and other pharmaceuticals which exploit the public's search for symptomatic medicines and undermine their independence and confidence in home remedies or traditional support systems which are often safer. An honourable and scientific profession cannot be seen to collude inadvertently with the commercialisation of normally self-limiting problems without ultimate denigration in the eyes of a better and better informed public. The error could not happen if clinicians considered population help-seeking patterns in addition to the conventional clinical process when managing their patients' problems; a desire to strengthen the public's resourcefulness and health should be the objective of every consultation in PHC because the moulding of future self-help practices is always an important consideration.

Epidemic Distress

Many of those who work in PHC still perceive their role as providing a front-line on-demand treatment for sick people, but the evidence from analysis of help-seeking patterns suggests that the degree of distress felt is much more important than the actual state of health in determining the use of PHC by individuals (Hulka et al. 1972; Kohn and White 1976). Distress is subjective and governed by many factors other than disease, particularly by the person's expectations, and thresholds of tolerance and social pressures. Expectations and fears are beginning to be recognised as powerful influences in epidemics of help seeking fuelled by social inadequacy, loss of self-confidence and rising claims from advertisers and experts that "someone else can do the job better than you".

The cough that is carelessly called whooping cough has been known to start an epidemic of pseudo-whooping cough by fanning the flames of fear in mothers and friends around the index case. Every cough then becomes:
"Whooping cough doctor?".

The well child with "earache last night" is often brought by a mother who can see that her child is fine, but for some reason she is unable to believe it — unable to use her maternal common sense in case she is blamed for being wrong or careless: "the doctor knows best" is a double-edged sword.

The clinician who is not willing to consider the impact of his work on patient's behaviour can fall easily into the Area-B trap of creating inappropriate help seeking (as in the pseudo-whooping cough example) and causes untold distress for patients and unnecessary work for himself and colleagues. Unfortunately, even some self-help manuals are becoming an ill-health growth industry and many are written by people with more common fear than common sense. It is safer for an author to be over-cautious because he cannot know his readers' abilities and an intended self-help manual can become referral guidelines or a set of rather muted information sheets with relevance to a small sector of the population.

There are, of course, the meek, disadvantaged or asymptomatic members of society who have serious problems which remain hidden to the PHC services because individuals are unaware, too timid or too disabled to demand attention — help seeking can be insufficient as well as excessive and every health care professional has a responsibility to attempt to achieve some degree of balance between expressed and unexpressed needs and the resources. Unfortunately, the complexity of these issues often leads clinicians to reject them as insoluble or capricious, but the developing principles of help-seeking behaviour and the practice of its modification are becoming important aspects of the discipline of PHC. Patients' decisions about when to seek professional help will determine how early many diagnoses can be made, the work load imposed on health services, the volume of sickness certification in a community and the number of opportunities for continuing care (Chap. 3) and anticipatory care (Chap. 5).

The principles of help seeking applicable to hospital care will not be discussed in this chapter, but the increasing involvement of specialists in some aspects of PHC has brought problems which will be increasingly important in the future. Casualty departments, asthma units, obstetric units and other specialist sectors which encourage the public to bypass PHC will become progressively flooded by more and more people who do not need specialist attention if the interfaces discussed in the next section of this chapter are ignored (see also Fig. 4.1). Specialists need to be most concerned with the help-seeking behaviour of professionals in PHC, leaving the help-seeking problems of patients to those in PHC, except in very unusual circumstances because, without this discipline, specialist standards will fall and PHC capabilities will be undermined. The interfaces in Fig. 4.1 show a wedge of direct contact between the public and the hospital sector and yet a dominance of problems which never reach a professional person. A balance between proportions in the different sectors is crucial for health service stability.

Use of PHC Facilities

Patients will use the services provided by PHC for one of two basic motivations:

1) either they know what they want and go to collect it, or
2) they are worried and go for medical help.

This dichotomy between the two categories of demand in PHC is important because patients in the former group do not feel they want a professional assessment, they are seeking a provision or service (doctor = shopkeeper). Those in the latter group are concerned about a problem(s) which they need to discuss with the doctor or nurse to negotiate a possible solution or course of action (conventional consultation). Many patients use clinical consultations for both purposes simultaneously.

Mr J.J. (42 years) enters the doctor's consulting room and requests a prescription for "my pills" (antihypertensive). He does not sit and would leave without further ado if the doctor just writes a prescription. His expectation on this occasion is for a provision without assessment.

Contrast this expectation for provision of a service with the category of demand where professional assistance is being sought.

Mrs P.P. (21 years) enters with an overswaddled baby in her arms and tear staining on her cheeks "He has been screaming all night doctor and now he is refusing to feed ..."

Many doctors and nurses feel that most patients should fall into the category of seeking help and advice, whereas consultations in most societies often fall into the former group, particularly in a nationalised, insurance-based or subsidised health care system. Patients are often aware of how some doctors become exasperated by being told what to provide, so clinical interviews can become very complicated if the doctor approaches the problem as a consultation yet the patient is too tactful to state that it is for a provision. The image of being an on-demand provider of medication, certification, normal deliveries or some other aspect of health care is far less attractive or prestigious than that of being consulted for considered diagnoses and treatments and so tensions are bound to arise when a patient's expectations are somewhat different from the doctor's, unless the inevitable duality of the doctor's role has been accepted. Recognition of the determinants of help-seeking behaviour and the relationship between it and clinical behaviour can help the clinician in PHC develop a much more objective view of the tensions and pressures which face those in the front-line of health care. Some sociological analysts have placed much emphasis on the clinician's role as provider of a service with associated patient rights (Blaxter and Patterson 1982), but the medical profession is understandably cautious of this oversimplification of their dual role because the relationship between provider and consumer is very different from that between consultant and patient, not just in terms of prestige but also in terms of having sufficient authority to contain and manage many very stormy human crises with which clinicians necessarily become involved (see Chap. 6).

Use of PHC in the United Kingdom, where a comprehensive health service is accessible to all people without financial barriers, has shown surprisingly large geographic and interdoctor variation (Hicks 1976; Howie 1977).

1) Huge variations of consultation rates from place to place and doctor to doctor.
2) Equally large variation in home visiting but a steady decline in the mean number since 1960.
3) A tendency for list size and consultation rate to be inversely related.
4) Huge variation in telephone consultations, repeat prescribing and out-of-hours calls.
5) About one-fifth of patients generate over half the work.

Unfortunately, few studies have attempted to examine the huge variation in use of PHC in terms of patients' expectations, in particular to define the proportion who expect a "provision" and those who need to "consult". Stimson and Webb (1975) found some evidence of these tensions in their interviews with patients before and after going to the doctor, and they developed a linear model to highlight the importance of patients' expectations with regard to their backgrounds. Subsequently, Fitton and Acheson (1979) developed and refined these principles in their detailed study of 320 patients who were asked what they wanted the doctor to do and whether this was also what they had expected to happen. They found that the doctors studied tended to underestimate patients' expectations for prescriptions, certificates, examinations, investigations and explanation. This work showed that the doctor did not always submit to patient pressure to provide what was wanted and this was achieved without excessive resentment or hostility in the people concerned — 68% of patients found talking to their doctor was always easy.

Fitton and Acheson also provided case histories which illustrated how expectations can be re-negotiated and modified by appropriate techniques, but this was less likely to be achieved when an expectation was held very strongly: the most emotional reactions came from patients who were not given a tranquilliser they expected.

My observation of colleagues and registrars who have videotaped or audiotaped their conversations with patients is that re-negotiation of expectations is most likely to fail if the tone is negative or defensive:

"John has a minor throat infection Mrs Jones, but he does not need penicillin, just give him aspirin."

The tone is defensive and the doctor sounds as if he would almost prefer to give the penicillin but for some reason does not; the "just give him aspirin" is rather weak. Let us contrast this with an exchange for a similar problem:

John really is a very healthy boy Mrs Jones, he has got a mild infection but his own resistance should deal with that over the next few days. Extra fruit and fluids are always good and soothing but I'm sure that you have your own home remedies too.

High and Low Users?

The breakdown of PHC utilisation into high- and low-user groups has been the basis of many studies and judgements, some of which are summarised in Table 4.2. Great care has to be taken in the interpretation of such data as individual items do not necessarily hold for all age groups and many features are interdependent. For example, Banks et al. (1975) indicated difficulty in establishing any relationship between demand for medical care and a variety of social variables in 20–44-year-old women, and when Collins and Klein (1980) analysed the general household survey data in the United Kingdom they showed that the conventional association between frequent demand for PHC and low social class was a direct product of the higher morbidity experience in the lower social classes. A "stereotype trap" can operate which encourages clinicians to oversimplify clusters of characteristics in a population and thereby develop views which are less than appropriate for a caring profession. A high user of PHC services can become inappropriately stigmatised by receptionists, nurses and even doctors. For example, Blaxter and Paterson (1982) have alleged that some very disadvantaged families in Aberdeen have low consultation rates because mothers are worried that their interpretation of symptoms may not match the medical profession's and they fear being seen to consult too frequently.

Stacey (1980) has pointed out that patients or parents with ill children can feel considerable anxiety about when it is appropriate to seek help over illness because doctors and nurses do not always take them sufficiently seriously, yet they also get blamed if they call for help too late. This "double-bind" situation was summed up by a mother who said "I'm either a careless parent or an over-anxious mum" — either way she was wrong and expressed feelings of frustration and helplessness in the face of a medical machine which she did not

Table 4.2. Characteristics of polar groups by frequency of attendance for PHC*

Feature	Frequent attender	Infrequent attender
1) Sex	More female	More male
2) Marital state	More single or divorced	More married
3) Age	Extremes of life often	Middle aged often
4) Social class	More in lower groups	More in upper groups
5) Physical diseases	Common	Less common
6) Neuroticism scores	Higher	Lower
7) Recent stress	More likely	Less likely
8) Self-image	More negative	More positive
9) Anxiety	Higher	Lower
10) Vulnerability feelings	Higher	Lower
11) Self-reliance	Lower	Higher
12) Economic problems	More	Fewer
13) Social problems	More	Fewer
14) Medical record size	Fat	Thin
15) Allegiance to doctor	Changed more often	Stable
16) Psychotropic medication	Common	Less common
17) Number in practice population	Few	Many
18) Social networks	Weak	Strong

*Sources: White et al. (1961); Balint (1964); Kessel and Shepherd (1965); Taylor (1968); Bice and White (1969); Polliack (1971); Wadsworth et al. (1971); Hulka (1972); McKinlay (1973); Hood and Farmer (1974); Bain and Philip (1975); Banks et al. (1975); Stimson and Webb (1975); Forster (1976); Hicks (1976); Anderson et al. (1977); Howie (1977); Mechanic (1978); Wolinsky (1978); Fitton and Acheson (1979); Otto (1979); Journal of the Royal College of General Practitioners (1982).

understand and which she felt had failed to comprehend her problems.

Taylor's view that less than 25% of the population cause over 50% of the work (Taylor 1954) is an oft-quoted statistic which can be interpreted to mean either that the high utilisers are a nuisance or that they need to be considered a special-needs group which requires specific strategies for its problems. There is certainly growing evidence in Europe that those in the high-user group are more likely to be ill, to have broken social networks and to be the products of industrial pressures which demand rehousing and high mobility (McKinlay 1973). The interpretation of utilisation of PHC services is further complicated by the fact there is controversy about whether individuals who use the services frequently cluster in the same families. Huygen (1978), in the Netherlands, found that family members resembled each other in consulting pattern, but others have found high-user families and high-user individuals often to be independent of one another (Wolinsky 1978). There is, of course, no necessary connection between disease and consultation rates, because PHC deals more with distress than with disease in all parts of the world and the conquest of many diseases has not always resulted in the conquest of distress.

Help seeking, as judged by utilisation rates, is obviously a very complex affair and it is fraught with the danger of simplistic generalisations and judgements. The data which are presented here suggest that the individual clinician would do well to remember that there is abundant evidence for both

50

sociodemographic factors and doctor/nurse behaviour as being determinants of patient's decisions to seek help. The clinician will have little control over the former, except through media propaganda and political action, whereas many opportunities occur every day to consider whether patients' problems are being handled in a way which will encourage each one to make appropriate use of the PHC services in the future. Cook-book practices which appear to collude with pharmaceutical company exploitation of the public's illness beliefs can only lead to a rising tide of expectations and eventual failures which may engulf and render impotent the front-line services. To operate successfully, PHC has to encourage patients to use available services appropriately and thereby strengthen lay networks and traditional home-healing practices which have kept 75% of symptoms outside PHC for generations (see Fig. 4.1).

Clinicians will sometimes be able to help to modify existing self-care practices in a useful way, e.g. avoidance of hypertonic infant feeds, saline purges or other dangerous home remedies, but the greater danger probably lies in making sweeping generalisations about these occasional errors and in tampering with independence and self-esteem so the medical role comes to dominate and create dependency just where it should be facilitating independence and family resourcefulness. Confident and capable mothers and fathers are a far greater asset to society than a sophisticated medical machine, and the modern discipline of PHC is just beginning to grasp this nettle and modify its practices accordingly.

Help Seeking and its Modification: Concluding Examples

The purpose of this chapter has been to review many of the factors which are important when individuals make their decisions to seek help from PHC services. The alert and well-trained clinician will consider every management plan against this background and an attempt has been made to show that many conventional medical managements are inappropriate when judged in this way. "What is appropriate therapy in traditional medical practice may be quite inappropriate if cognisance is taken of patient's confidence and future help seeking" — this approach should cast fresh light on every treatment plan. Many of the case examples have involved individual patients because this is how clinicians make most of their decisions, but some PHC academics have applied group (campaign) methods instead.

Marsh (1977) mounted a concerted campaign in his group practice to reduce the public's dependency for minor ailments. Doctors, nurses, health visitors and receptionists advertised a policy of not prescribing for self-limiting minor complaints. Instead self-care using home remedies was encouraged. He reported a great fall in the number of consultations for minor ailments and the local pharmacists experienced a similar decline in business for cough mixtures, diarrhoeal mixtures and analgesics, etc. Cartwright's (1979) anxiety that this policy would produce adverse effects on the population was not born out, the public expressing satisfaction with the service despite the change of policy.

An example of population education was evaluated at the Department of General Practice, St Thomas's Hospital Medical School, where a randomised controlled trial of an information booklet describing the management of common problems for literate patients led to a significant shift towards self-care for the relevant problems (Anderson et al. 1980; Morrell et al. 1980). The behaviour change was not, however, related to improved theoretical knowledge in the experimental group. Marsh (1980) likewise found that a practice brochure was highly acceptable to patients and helped to shift demand for family planning and minor trauma to the practice nurse as well as improving the patients' perception of teamwork in the practice.

The virtual conquest of severe malnutrition in a Zulu community over a period of 10–15 years has been attributed to a programme of nutrition education integrated with PHC and a productive home-garden development which enabled the rural people to choose their food more wisely, prepare their food with less destruction of nutrients and, for some, to use their small garden for the local production of essential nutrients (Stott 1976). The health consequences of this broad and integrated approach have been impressive (Fig. 4.3) and the fostering of independence from charity is an important feature of the sociomedical project which is relevant to both help seeking and the opportunistic health care described in Chapter 5. Newell (1975) has endorsed the principle of self-help and resourcefulness in his review of ten other innovative community health schemes and, despite the short-term benefits of food fortification and supplementation programmes in the less developed areas, most experienced community health workers now acknowledge the long-term dangers of propping people up in nutritional terms because they never learn to make appropriate independent choices which can have a lasting impact on community health (McNaughton 1975; Sevenhuysen and Burgess 1980).

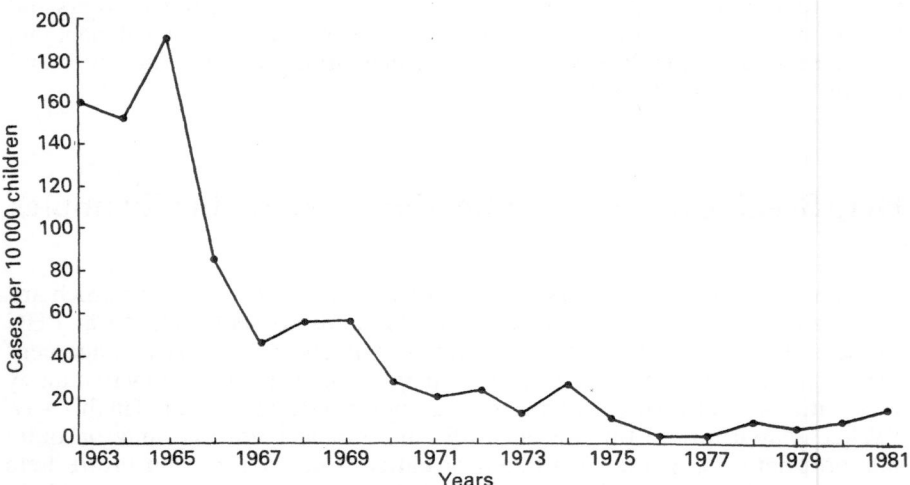

Fig. 4.3. Decline of kswashiorkor associated with an integrated sociomedical approach to the community. The graph shows the number of cases of kwashiorkor per 10 000 children aged 0–7 attending clinic. (The Valley Trust Annual Report 1981.)

Perhaps the biggest pharmaceutically designed and uncontrolled experiment ever to be conducted on help seeking is the massive shift in public expectations and behaviours concerning psychotropic drugs. The staggering international increase in use of antidepressants and tranquillisers has been largely independent of national and political differences (Kohn and White 1976). That most people still avoid psychopharmacology for psychic distress (Lancet 1978) is an indication of the potential for a further landslide in the direction of drug use (Koumjian 1981) and pressure on the prescribers unless those in PHC examine the efficacy of psychopharmaceutical preparations in terms of future help-seeking behaviour and interpersonal skills (Kessel 1979) in addition to conventional clinical criteria. There is now overwhelming evidence that the modification of feelings of distress is not always a humane clinical response because the consequences can be a devastating dependence on drug treatment for every life crisis (Kohn and White 1976; Lancet 1978; Koumjian 1981), the value of short-term relief being traded for the danger of a "pill response" to stress.

Appropriate preventive care should, of course, reduce the need for medical crisis intervention; the reduction in asthmatic crises at night being an example of secondary prevention, and good antenatal care being an example of clinical primary prevention. However, both these familiar examples probably result in more routine attendances and a greater overall number of attendances for PHC services for monitoring. True reductions in help seeking are most likely to come from conditions which do not need continuing care, those which are totally preventable (see Chap. 5), and those which the patient/family can redefine as problems for self-care or lay control. Increases in help seeking which may merit our attention are to be found among patients who are old and undemanding and others who suffer social disadvantage in silence. Even adolescents sometimes need to be encouraged to consult because their reticence can be a barrier to availing themselves of help. Yet in these theoretical risk groups, there is often honour and pride in independence and the PHC clinician who interferes with this treasure without invitation or very good reason will be guilty of damage to the fabric of society and meddlesome medicalisation unless as a fully accepted member of the community.

Unfortunately, many students do not progress beyond a limited understanding of help seeking (Area B) and many teachers still do not insist on rigorous application of the principles. To ask whether each intervention or management plan takes cognisance of future help seeking is one of the disciplines in PHC which needs wider recognition, and so a hand-out for the guidance of inexperienced teachers in undergraduate PHC is included in Appendix II. This hand-out is intended as a quick and easy reference source to stimulate the teaching of a more disciplined and comprehensive approach to PHC during day-to-day clinical work. It was written and used in the Welsh National School of Medicine but the principles are generally applicable, even if some of the examples are culturally specific to Wales.

References

Anderson JAD, Buck D, Danaher KM, Fry J (1977) Users and non-users of doctors — implication for self-care. J Roy Coll Gen Pract 27:155–160

Anderson JE, Morrell DC, Avery AJ, Watkins CJ (1980) Evaluation of a patient education manual. Br Med J 281:924–926

Bain DJG, Philip AE (1975) Going to see the doctor — attendances by members of 100 families in their first year in a new town. J Roy Coll Gen Pract 25:821–827

Baker CD (1976) Non-attenders in general practice. J Roy Coll Gen Pract 26:404–409

Balint M (1964) The doctor, his patient and the illness. Pitman Medical, London

Banks M, Beresford D, Morrell D, Waller J, Watkins C (1975) Factors influencing demand for primary medical care in women aged 20–44 years. Intern J Epidemiol 4:189–195

Bice TW, White KL (1969) Factors related to the use of health services — an international comparative study. Med Care 7:124–133

Blaxter M, Paterson E (1982) Mothers and daughters. A three-generation study of health attitudes and behaviour. Heinemann, London

Blumhagen D (1980) Hypertension: a folk illness with a medical name. Culture, Med Soc 4:197–227

Cartwright Anne (1979) Minor illness in the surgery. In: McCarthy M (ed) Management of minor illness. King Edward's Hospital Fund, London, pp 11–21

Collins E, Klein R (1980) Equity and the NHS: self-reported morbidity, access and primary care. Br Med J 281:1111–1115

Cosminsky S (1975) Changing food and medical beliefs and practices in a Guatemalan community. Ecol Food Nutr 4:183–191

Crombie DL, Pinsent RJFH, Lambert DM, Birch D (1975) Comparison of first and second national morbidity surveys. J Roy Coll Gen Pract 25:874–878

Danaher K (1979) Education for self-care. In: McCarthy M (ed) Management of minor illness. King Edward's Hospital Fund, London, pp 69–86

Elliott-Binns CP (1973) An analysis of lay medicine. J Roy Coll Gen Pract 23:255–264

Fitton F, Acheson HWK (1979) The doctor–patient relationship. HMSO, London

Forster DP (1976) Social class differences in sickness and GP consultation. Health Trends 8:29–32

Helman C (1978) Feed a cold, starve a fever — folk models of infection in an English suburban community. Culture, Med Soc 2:107–137

Hicks D (1976) Primary health care. HMSO, London

Hood JE, Farmer R (1974) A comparative study of frequent and infrequent attenders at a general practice. Intern J Nursing Studies 11:147–153

Horder J, Horder E (1954) Illness in general practice. Practitioner 173:177–187

Howie JGR (1977) Patterns of work. In: Fry J (ed) Trends in general practice. British Medical Journal Press, London, pp 22–35

Hulka B, Kuppar LL, Cassell JC (1972) Determinants of physician utilisation. Med Care 10:300–309

Huygen FJA (1978) Family medicine. Dekker and Van de Vegt, Nijmegen

Illich I (1977) Medical nemesis: the expropriation of health. Pelican, London

Journal of the Royal College of General Practitioners (1982) Editorial. J Roy Coll Gen Pract 32:396–397

Katz AH (1979) Self-help health groups. Soc Sci Med 13A:491–494

Kennedy I (1980) The Reith lectures. BBC, London

Kessel N (1979) Reassurance. Lancet i:1128–1133

Kessel N, Shepherd M (1965) The health and attitudes of people who seldom consult a doctor. Med Care 3:6–10

Kleinman A (1979) Patients and healers in the context of culture. University of California Press, Berkeley

Kohn R, White KL (eds) (1976) Health care — an international study. Oxford University Press, London

Koumjian K (1981) The use of Valium as a form of social control. Soc Sci Med 15E:245–249

Lancet (1978) Stress, distress and drug treatment (editorial). Lancet ii:1347–1348

Locker D (1981) Symptoms and illness. The cognitive organisation of disorder. Tavistock, London

Mabry JH (1964) Lay concepts of etiology. J Chron Dis 17:371–386

McKinlay JB (1973) Social networks, lay consultation, help-seeking behaviour. Soc Forces 51(3):275–292

McNaughton J (1975) Applied nutrition programmes. The past as a guide for the future. Food Nutr 1(3): 17–23

Marsh GN (1977) Curing minor illness in general practice. Br Med J 2:1267–1269

Marsh GN (1980) The practice brochure: a patient's guide to team care. Br Med J 281:730–732

Mechanic D (1978) Effects of psychological distress on perception of physical health and use of medical psychiatric facilities. J Human Stress 4:26–32

Melville A (1980) Job satisfaction in general practice: implications for prescribing. Soc Sci Med 14A:495–499

Morrell DC, Avery AJ, Watkins CJ (1980) The management of minor illness. Br Med J 280:769–771

Newell KW (1975) Health by the people. WHO, Geneva

Office of Home Economics (1975) Health care dilemma or "Am I Kranken, doctor?" Office of

Home Economics, London

Otto R (1979) Negative and positive life experience among men and women in selected occupations, symptom awareness and visits to the doctor. Soc Sci Med 13A:151–164

Pill R, Stott NCH (1982) Concepts of illness causation and responsibility: some preliminary data from a sample of working class mothers. Soc Sci Med 16:43–52

Polliack MR (1971) The relationship between Cornell Medical Index scores and attendance rates. J Roy Coll Gen Pract 21:453

Sevenhuysen GP, Burgess AP (1980) Evaluation of nutrition interventions. An annotated bibliography and review of methodologies and results. ESN/MISC/80/4. FAO, UNO, Rome

Stacey M (1978) Sociological concepts of health and disease and critiques of such concepts. SSRC Symposium, Sheffield

Stacey M (1980) Realities for change in child health care: existing patterns and future possibilities. Br Med J 280:1512–1515

Stimson C, Webb B (1975) In: Going to see the doctor. Routledge and Kegan Paul, London, pp 28–33

Stott HH (1976) The Valley Trust socio-medical project for the promotion of health in a less developed rural area. MD Thesis, University of Edinburgh

Taylor PJ (1968) Personal factors associated with sickness absence. Br J Indust Med 25:106

Taylor S (1954) Good general practice. British Medical Association, London, p 420

Wadsworth MEJ, Butterfield WJH, Blaney R (1971) Health and sickness: the choice of treatment. Tavistock, London

White KL, Williams TF, Greenberg BG (1961) The ecology of medical care. NZ J Med 265:885–892

Wilson JL (1977) Family utilisation of a medical centre. J Fam Pract 5:991–996

Wolinsky FD (1978) Assessing the effects of predisposing, enabling and illness-morbidity characterisation on health service utilisation. J Health Soc Behaviour 19:384–396

Young JC (1980) A model of illness decisions in a Tarascan town. Am Ethnol 7:1006–1031

5. Primary Opportunistic and Anticipatory Health Care

No longer is it necessary to defend the importance of prevention in health care. Successive international and local reports from many sources have recognised the importance of promoting health and preventing disease (Lalonde 1974; Mayer and Sainsbury 1975; Newell 1975; Consultative Document 1976; Barr and Logan 1977; Royal College of General Practitioners 1981; Alma Ata Declaration — see Appendix I.) Neither is there much dispute about the value of most basic statutory methods to improve public health; clean water, clean air, sanitation and regulation of food handlers are either taken for granted by those who have them or sought after by those who do not have them. However, differences of opinion do arise in two important aspects of prevention.

1) The role of PHC professionals in consumer motivation for health and prevention of illness.
2) The role of PHC in looking for undiagnosed or asymptomatic problems.

The framework described in this book (see Fig. 2.1) emphasises the concept of opportunistic prevention in PHC because every contact with patients provides opportunities for the prevention of illness and the encouragement of people to adopt more healthy life-styles, even when the patient has come for an apparently unrelated problem which has to be dealt with first. In this chapter, it shall be argued that this is part of the modern discipline of PHC and that it is a highly professional manner of working which integrates curative, caring and preventive work with individuals yet encourages most people to remain responsible for their own health.

The emphasis in opportunistic health care is on taking the opportunities offered by patients. An alternative term which is widely used and very descriptive is "anticipatory care"; here the emphasis is on anticipating patients' future problems and trying to prevent them from occurring. The latter term was probably coined by Van den Dool (1970) following a large multiphasic screening project of 4000 patients in a Netherlands' rural general practice. He concluded that population screening was an inappropriate activity for PHC because it was wasteful and failed to make use of the natural advantages of the PHC setting. He favoured the opportunistic use of every patient contact to achieve basic observations and early diagnoses without resort to specific population screening, and he called this anticipatory care. Tudor Hart (1975) has echoed this view and provided abundant evidence for the efficacy of opportunistic diagnosis of hypertension in his Welsh general practice, and Sackett and Holland (1975) have coined the term "case-finding" to demonstrate the way PHC doctors can already identify and treat the more vulnerable members of the population during day-to-day consultations. Morrell (1978) has emphasised that the team which makes the diagnosis must also be responsible for continuing care or there is risk of patients being picked up but not treated. Furthermore, special screening teams have a high probability of diagnosing disorders which are already known to the patients' general practitioners — a wasteful duplication of effort and an indication that well-organised PHC should not need external mass screening exercises.

However, the opportunities provided in every PHC consultation for anticipatory action are not confined to early diagnosis and treatment; it is increasingly evident that the choices people make over their food, their habits, their relationships and activities can all have an impact on future health and the one-to-one contacts between doctor/nurse and members of the public are important opportunities for these issues to be raised with tact and diplomacy. This "personal health education" is a delicate area for negotiation because the doctor/nurse may be commenting on life-style decisions and patterns which are highly personal and idiosyncratic, and the patient has every right to resent this as interference unless it is introduced with sensitivity, bearing in mind that it is usually some other problem that brought the patient to PHC (Stott 1981). The role of the clinician in opportunistic health care is totally different from the conventional role in dealing with presenting and continuing problems because use is made of the opportunity provided by the consultation to try to encourage the patient/family to modify a potentially dangerous life-style which may even be cherished or enjoyed. A caring clinician cannot accept slow self-destruction in people seen professionally, however much they may enjoy the habits, without some attempt to provide help; but neither can compliance be expected if the style of life has been chosen with full awareness of the risks.

Mr J.J. (32 years) saw Dr P. regularly for hypertension management but he showed no interest in Dr P.'s attempts to help him lose weight and stop smoking — he said he "enjoyed excessive eating, drinking and fags so much that he had no desire to change".

The Feldstein family, who also attended Dr P.'s health centre, were heavy smokers until their first child was born prematurely. Discussion about the possible causes of this event and some skilled help and support from a health visitor led to a radical change in the family's dietary habits as well as complete success over stopping smoking.

Mrs L.P. had taken her child twice to the teaching hospital 30 miles away where he had been admitted with severe malnutrition, cured and returned to her poor home on an African hillside where the staple diet was refined mealie-meal porridge. Poverty was one barrier to health but a PHC team who helped her to use the soil around her home to grow food supplements was far more relevant to her permanent needs and independence than the dramatic cures of the paediatric wing of the hospital and the advice of successive clinic doctors.

These brief anecdotes illustrate how conventional medical practice has to be modified if the needs of people are to be met in terms of opportunistic health promotion at a level acceptable to the patient. In the first case history, Dr P. had to accept the risks his patient chose and provide conventional supervision to control his hypertension (secondary prevention). In the second case, Dr P. enlisted the aid of his health visitor to help the Feldsteins through a difficult time caring for a premature infant. Both the doctor and the health visitor encouraged them to review their "junk-food" dietary habits and to use a simple programme for smoking reduction. The family proved to be very receptive to this practical approach to reducing the risks in the next pregnancy. The final example of an African child on the revolving door of malnutrition in and out of hospital is taken from an account of a unique experiment among the Zulu. A PHC clinic was extended by a nutrition education unit, agricultural demonstration unit and field extension work, so extremely poor Zulu mothers could learn to use the resources around them (the soil) and produce food supplements locally as well as learn about cooking, food preparation practices and environmental rehabilitation to produce a lasting impact on their families' health and quality of life (The Valley Trust Annual Reports 1954–1982; Stott 1959, 1973, 1976).

Opportunism in health care is using the opportunities people give to those in PHC to help them (the patients) build on their assets: if they are too affluent, they may be choosing destructive life-styles and if they have too little, they can feel more trapped in unhealthy life-styles than they need to be. In both situations the clinician can sometimes help if PHC is organised to respond in innovative ways and if clinicians are prepared to be very practical and specific.

Three Sources of Innovation

The Peckham Experiment (London).
A Review of Ten Innovative Community Health Schemes (Multinational).
The Valley Trust Sociomedical Experiment (Kwa-Zulu).

Each of these sources has approached the problems of community health in diverse cultural situations and each has influenced the development of the principle of opportunism in PHC. The Peckham Experiment (Pearce and Crocker 1944) was mounted in London in the 1930s and was closed down at the advent of the National Health Service. An unusual "health centre" consisted of inner-city indoor recreation facilities such as swimming bath, badminton, boxing, tennis, table-tennis, snack bar, coffee bar, etc., a medical service run by doctors, nurses and scientists and close links with a farm on the outskirts of London. In pre-war London, poverty, poor housing and lack of primary health care for common ailments had resulted in a massive amount of preventable ill-health. The project was based upon family subscription and it represented an attempt to encourage East-end families to learn to choose good food, habits and recreational activities which would enhance family health in the broadest sense. Families could choose to join the centre and to use the opportunities it provided for discovery of healthy life-styles, particularly in relation to hygiene, exercise, nutrition, relationships and family bonds. The director of the Peckham Experiment found a huge amount of undiagnosed or subclinical disorder which was readily amenable to either life-style modification or treatment. The project represented a synthesis of recreation facilities, diagnostic facilities and educational opportunities and (good) food availability in a megalopolis; it was a rare and remarkable fore-runner of an integrated and positive approach to health promotion, but it was closed by the advent of the National Health Service because it did not fit into any of the established ministries of the day. The scientists and clinicians working in

Peckham perceived every family problem as an opportunity to kindle and encourage healthy life-styles, including consumption of fresh farm produce in the centre of London in the 1930s!

In less developed countries, the basic problems of community health are similar in their origins to those of pre-war London, but different in their manifestations and potential for improvement. Innovative experiments have been reported which illustrate how food, education and productivity in poor areas can have a considerable impact on people's health in the absence of highly technical and procedural medical care. Projects have been described by authors from China, Cuba, Guatemala, India, Indonesia, Iran, Niger, Tanzania and Venezuela, and these are well reviewed by Newell (1975) who showed how involvement of the local community is a key to people's successful participation in preventive and promotive health. The diverse schemes were all remarkable for the sense of community responsibility and involvement, for individual and group self-sufficiency, and for the "feeling that people have a true unity between their land, their work and their household". Newell's major regret was that most evaluations of these schemes had been very short term or limited by scarce resources.

A sociomedical experiment which was not included in Newell's book but which has nearly 30 years of well-documented progress is the rural Valley Trust project among the Zulu. Alarmingly high levels of malnutrition after the Second World War stimulated the founder to combine a rural health centre, nutrition education, health-garden promotion and wider recreational and social activities in a practical, patient-and-community-involving exercise which pioneered the principle of opportunism in PHC. The clinician became a motivator towards practical food choices and food production in addition to performing a curative role. This was made possible by the creation of a "referral chain" from clinic to nutrition education area to agricultural demonstration and to home-based fieldwork, and it has led to a decline in the occurrence of kwashiorkor (protein–calorie malnutrition) in the area, a decline which became steepest in the second decade of the project and has remained low (see Fig. 4.4). Evidence that this decline has been due to community participation in the nutritional and sociomedical approach to ill-health is well documented in successive annual reports (The Valley Trust Annual Reports 1954–1982) and a thesis (Stott 1976) which illustrates how surrounding areas, which were less influenced by the Trust's activities, have continued to experience serious malnutrition throughout the 25 years studied.

The importance of personal responsibility for health and patient participation in their PHC was firmly declared by the 1978 World Health Organisation Alma-Ata Conference (Appendix I). But it seems that the less developed countries are more likely to implement the aims of that conference, which emphasised the role of opportunistic PHC, preventive medicine and community development in its most basic participatory forms. Newell (1975) himself said that none of the ten schemes he reported separated promotional, preventive or curative services at the primary care level and he was highly critical of sectorisation in health matters: "a strict health sectorial approach is ineffective, other actions outside the field of health perhaps having greater health effects than strictly health care interventions". His summary of the order of priorities in the ten schemes was:

1) Social and economic injustice
2) Land tenure
3) Agriculture and marketing
4) Population control
5) Malnutrition
6) Health training
7) Curative medicine

This hierarchy of priorities is a reflection of the emphasis Newell placed on different aspects of health. In the light of his review, however, it is interesting that in many of the schemes, simple PHC was used as one of the entry points into a complex social system without upsetting the existing structures or resourcefulness of the indigenous people. This principle of facilitating change towards more healthy life-styles without the destruction of pride and independence is almost unheard of in affluent nations and yet is was well demonstrated in The Valley Trust project and restated by many of the authors in Newell's review.

How can others in PHC work towards some of the principles shown in these innovative community projects? Simple advice or counselling about health will seldom be enough unless it is very practical and specific, and it is likely that progressive PHC will become more and more concerned with approaches which may be initiated in the consulting room but which will certainly not stop there. The number of patients attending PHC of their own volition and the fact that many of them come for advice/help, render the PHC situation an exceptionally suitable one for initiating change towards healthier life-style choices or appropriate early diagnostic techniques, but these will need to be fashioned to the individual's needs and adapted on successive contacts which may sometimes occur in patients' homes. Those in PHC who are prepared and able to develop more opportunistic anticipatory care in their work will need to do so against background knowledge of:

1) the antecedents of health behaviours;
2) the levels of opportunistic anticipatory care;
3) skills and practices in opportunistic anticipatory care;
4) priorities for anticipatory care in each area.)

1) The Antecedents of Health Behaviours

The determinants of behaviour and choices are a very complex subject and the numerous factors involved are summarised in the cascade diagram (Fig. 5.1). Not all behaviours are logical or considered, some are habits or family patterns, some are results of frustrated attempts to change and some are bad because people are motivated by harmful as well as healthy things. The barriers to change can also be considerable: poverty, weakness, disability, fear, disinterest, religion, negativism, jealousy, greed, education, etc. can all stand in the way of change. The most widely known and researched scheme to provide a

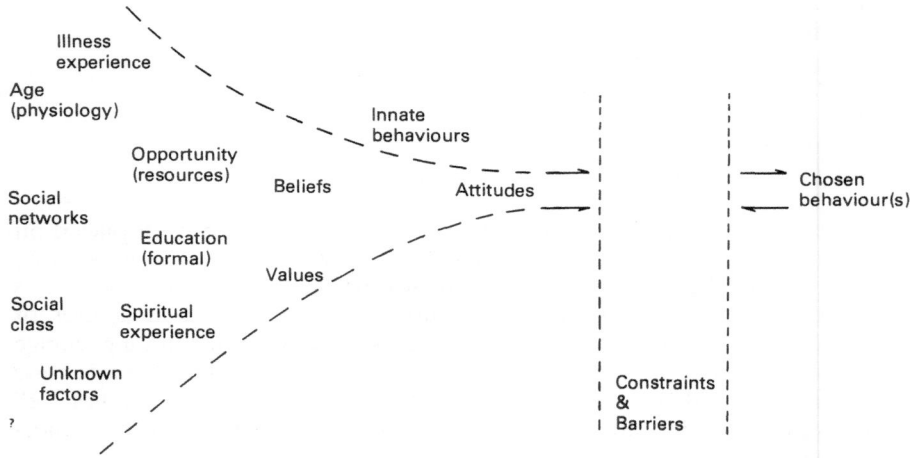

Fig. 5.1. Cascade of factors influencing an individual's health and illness behaviour.

theoretical understanding about how people come to their choices which influence health is the "health belief model" (HBM) (Rosenstock 1974; Becker et al. 1977). This states that an action a person takes for the purpose of preventing disease is largely determined by:

1) how susceptible they feel to a disorder;
2) how seriously the disorder is perceived;
3) a weighing-up of the advantages of prevention versus the cost (human and financial) of the proposed change/choice;
4) the general health motivation of the individual;
5) any cues/trigger factors which tip the balance of the decision one way or another.

The HBM is a detailed consideration of factors near the apex of the cascade diagram (Fig. 5.1) and it is based largely on research into uptake by the public, of specific procedures and the early detection of diseases. However, the same principles probably apply to other life-style choices *if* the individual has a general motivation for maintenance of health. Unfortunately, this is not always true and it seems that a significant proportion of people are very fatalistic about their ability to have any control/choice over future health and illness (Stott and Pill 1980; Pill and Stott 1982); others make many decisions by accident. Responses to health education are not necessarily logical and an element of the unpredictable is usually present. One explanation for this is that the search for recognition and the hunger for emotional, physical and psychological intimacy are drives which are so powerful that they will override many logical thoughts (Berne 1966). Others have suggested that the desire for spiritual experience is an equal or greater overriding factor: for example, three themes which provide anchors between belief and behaviour were described by Vaux (1976) in his review of religion and health as:

1) a goal of purity in life (clean living);
2) a goal of peace in existence (peace);
3) a belief in immortality (health and life for ever).

Each of these was considered to influence health attitudes and behaviour and all three are common to most religions. An active religious allegiance has been correlated with fewer physical and mental symptoms (Hannay 1980), and Durkheim (1951) has shown that an active religion does protect the individual against some of the hazards of urban living, but research on the subject is limited.

> The increase of smoking in young Western women was interpreted by Vaux to be a manifestation of the search for peace through autonomy and experience but only achieved by placing less importance on inner purity (cigarettes are dirty) and immortality (the young are always less concerned with this aspect).

Motives and meaning obviously become very important when we search to understand the reasons for people's choices for themselves or their families in illness (see Chap. 4) and in health. A cascade of factors interact and summate towards a final common pathway in health decisions (Fig. 5.1), but this summary diagram can only help us begin to understand the individual because personal priorities and values modify both the power and direction of the cascade forces and many barriers can inhibit the implementation of intellectual or instinctive desires. It is most unlikely that we will ever predict health behaviour with precision, but the clinician in PHC can only provide care in an informed way if aware and interested in those pressures and fears which make some decisions about health difficult or impossible. Only then will clinicians stop offering facile advice, facile not because of its content but because of lack of insight into the barriers which prevent the patient from following the words of professional wisdom.

> You have no idea how rude that doctor was to me . . . he tore a strip off me for not losing weight . . . I thought I must have gained 2½ stone but you know what I have gained . . . 2½ pounds! (laughs) . . . I suppose I have to take him with a pinch of salt because the poor fellow is foreign and he just doesn't understand my problems. (Welsh patient after visit to a metabolic clinic.)

It will come as no surprise to know that this patient defaulted from the next two follow-up clinics in the metabolic unit and an irate letter eventually arrived on her family physician's desk from the specialist in metabolic diseases:

> Dear Dr S.
>
> *Mrs P. (38)*
>
> This patient has defaulted from my clinic on three occasions and so I presume that she no longer wishes to attend for treatment. When last seen she had gained 2½ pounds and seemed poorly motivated to adhere to her diet.

Who, may we ask, was poorly motivated? The patient who had not performed as expected or the doctor who had not behaved as expected? To be rude to Mrs P. implied that she was to blame and needed sharp correction, but this was unlikely to be a useful tactic because Mrs P. perceived her problem in a different light (she felt that she had "gland trouble" which the metabolic specialist would fix and, having discovered that he had no special skills, she dropped him).

Suggestions for change in the choices people make are only likely to be noted or followed if the person concerned feels that the clinician is sensitive to the reasons for behaving in a particular way. This is partly achieved by good interview technique (see Chap. 1), but it also depends on awareness of those issues which are difficult to change in the person's background. Only then will it be possible for the PHC clinician to help the person to plan a practical and empathetic approach to the problem(s).

In the absence of background information, the clinician is likely to be insensitive to the perceptions and pressures depicted in Fig. 5.1 and be liable to draw poor compliance (Becker et al. 1979), negative reactions from patients and loss of confidence in professional help.

2) Levels of Opportunistic Anticipatory Care

The diversity of standards of training and practice in PHC means that it is necessary for teachers and clinicians to consider three categories of anticipatory care which also illustrate varying degrees of organisational and individual complexity.

0) No anticipatory PHC practised.
1) Ad hoc anticipatory PHC.
2) Systematic anticipatory PHC.

0) In the "zero category" no attempt is made by clinicians to practise anticipatory care. They work with presenting and continuing morbidity alone, sometimes taking cognisance of help-seeking patterns.

1) Ad hoc anticipatory care involves clinicians performing occasional screening tests or counselling about health habits procedures or even referral to other agencies. Ad hoc activity is quite common in PHC because most doctors will respond to some situations in an anticipatory way, particularly if a serious disease triggers them to think of it. Furthermore, so much publicity has surrounded some preventive activities (e.g. obesity, alcohol abuse, smoking) that even those who overeat, drink excessively, or smoke themselves, will advise patients to change a habit or put them in touch with an appropriate helping agency. Ad hoc anticipatory care is the most common form of prevention in PHC, particularly when education of patients about their diseases overlaps with teaching about risk factors which are modifiable, but too few PHC centres offer anything more than superficial advice.

Bartlett (1980), reviewing the contribution of PHC consumer health education in the United States, described four observational studies in which 19%–35% of consultation time was devoted to health education and counselling by doctors, but most of the work he quoted in his review dealt with conventional medical functions, such as compliance with therapy, appointment keeping, knowledge of diagnosis and understanding of therapy, which do not really qualify as anticipatory care because so many of these legitimate clinical activities are really part of the management of the presenting problem or continuing problems. Some truly anticipatory functions have, however, become a routine component of clinical examination; for example, cervical cytology in gynaecological practice, or advice about smoking habits in patients with chest diseases. Unfortunately, the number of items which are potentially available for anticipatory care is enormous and the weakness of the ad hoc approach is that the clinician can do what he feels like doing or is cued to do by the patient without any attempt to be systematic or disciplined. A patchy and incomplete coverage of anticipatory care is the inevitable outcome of the ad hoc approach, but at least any help given is likely to be perceived by the patient as relevant to the clinical problem.

2) Systematic anticipatory care implies that the clinician organises the approach to each patient to include a consideration of risk factors which may be relevant to future health of the individual or family. The realisation of this laudable aim is often frustrated because the time available is limited, the theoretical list of possibilities is large, records are often incomplete and ancillary back-up is often inadequate. It is essential, therefore, for priorities to be established for each patient and so highly selective but personally appropriate anticipatory care can be the result. This is often the best that can be achieved in an average PHC environment and it has the merit of being possible when team methods are out of the question for organisational reasons or when only one doctor/nurse in a group is ready to widen the scope of his or her professional work in this way.

Mrs P: "Peter is not feeding well and has been feverish overnight."
Dr Z: "Let me see . . . yes, he has a very red eardrum which needs treatment but I would also like to check it again in about 2 weeks as he seems rather rundown. Incidentally, I notice that he never had his full course of immunisation . . . was that by accident or design?"

In this example Dr Z. brought the child back for three reasons: overtly, to check his ear, but more important was the observation that Peter was rather thin and pale and looked small for his age, as well as having had incomplete immunisation.

Three factors contributed to the breadth of the above consultation.

1) The fact that Mrs P. brought Peter to PHC.
2) The doctor's willingness to look beyond the child's immediate problem and consider his observed size in relation to age as well as general clinical features and nutritional status.
3) A clinical record which revealed incomplete immunisation.

"Peter" was subsequently found to be malnourished and on the third percentile for weight and height, as well as suffering from severe dental decay, probably associated with multiple course of antibiotic syrups and a high-sucrose diet. His family had moved almost every 6 months since his birth due to housing difficulties. Clinical opportunism faced his mother with his nutritional problems, growth delay, recurrent (unnecessary) infections, poor dental status and need for diphtheria, tetanus and polio immunisation. Peter's illness also seemed to trigger his parents to reconsider their local situation and to settle for a less than perfect but much more stable home which was, perhaps, the most important factor in his continued development, because 2 years later his growth had returned to above the tenth percentile. Opportunistic analysis in the initial consultation was quick but it initiated work for the health visitor and practice nurse who helped the family achieve the targets described here by attention to food choices, child-rearing practices, immunisation and greater involvement of the father in household budgeting.

Antagonism to systematic anticipatory care has been expressed by some clinicians who confuse social help with social interference. For example, a doctor who also happened to know "Peter's" family commented that the health visitor had been a "social busybody trying to run the lives of others". He used this view to reject the principle of opportunism in PHC and we must consider whether this is valid criticism. The test for validity is quite simple: did the PHC team help the family to become more independent of the helping services or did the care lead to greater dependence on social and clinical support? In the example given, the former was true and the criticism of the principle of opportunism could not be upheld, but there always is a very thin dividing line between helping people to be independent of aid and making them dependent on aid. An oft-used quotation in The Valley Trust literature which captures this point is the Chinese proverb: "Give a man a fish and you feed him for one day, teach a man to fish and you feed him for ever" (The Valley Trust Annual Reports 1954–1982).

In Fig. 5.2, two organisational approaches to anticipatory care are depicted graphically, and in Table 5.1 their differences are compared. The "cohort method" and the "opportunistic method" are not mutually exclusive but they can be mutually wasteful and confusing if ill-coordinated. The traditional cohort method involves sending for a selected group of the population and offering them some aspect of anticipatory care, e.g. immunisation, developmental review, cervical cytology, preconception preparation, mother-

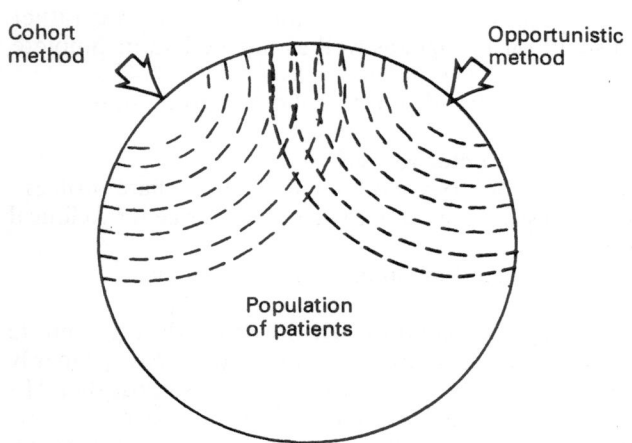

Fig. 5.2. Two approaches to anticipatory care: the impact of either a cohort or opportunistic approach to a population of people. (Note the potential for duplication of effort unless the two are co-ordinated.)

Table 5.1. Comparison of two systematic approaches to anticipatory care

	Systematic	
	Cohort method	Opportunistic method
Integrates prevention + cure	No	Yes
Specific recall of patients	Yes	Only occasional non-attenders at risk
Centralised records necessary	Yes	No but helpful
Personal records essential	No	Yes
Extra clinic necessary	Usually	No
Extra staff needed	Usually	Not usually
Postage costs	Yes	Minimal
Defaulters defined early	Yes, quickly	Over a longer period
Overall cost (financial)	High	Low
Accessibility for patient	Limited	Good
Job satisfaction (clinician)	Limited	Good
Paramedical involvement	Full	Partial

craft classes, blood pressure screening, etc. In the opportunistic method, the whole PHC team agrees to use most contacts with patients to check that their anticipatory care needs have been met and a personal medical record which doctor, nurse or patient keeps, reflects what has been achieved. Priorities are decided for each area and targets can be set for a population of patients which are compatible with the resources. A defined patient population is desirable for either approach.

The best of both methods should theoretically be possible if monitoring of anticipatory care is used to identify people who slip through the opportunistic PHC net so any reminders or invitations are only sent to a subgroup.

Where no comprehensive PHC service has developed, a fragmented cohort approach to anticipatory care is almost inevitable until several special clinics can be moulded into a disciplined PHC facility. The local health authority clinics in Great Britain are an example of specialised clinics which have been run by well-trained staff to achieve family planning, immunisation and developmental assessments on children, but their importance is waning as the PHC services become better able to embrace most anticipatory functions. Similarly, many maternal and child health clinics in less developed countries provide some basic anticipatory care for mothers and children because no comprehensive PHC exists (Edstrom 1979; Scotney 1979). However, these clinics usually grow to provide much more than their specific aims — they begin to provide integrated PHC to mothers and children but eschew the wider responsibilities of PHC in other age groups.

Those who run PHC services have to decide whether they will perpetuate the traditional cohort approach with increasing numbers of special clinics or build an opportunistic method which is less familiar to those whose training has been dominated by specialists. A difficulty experienced by clinicians is that they are usually taught about diseases and cohorts of people with certain characteristics — a tidy disorder-specific and reductionist discipline which bears little relationship to the way people appear in PHC. Patients come at critical moments with varied and often multiple problems and only the appropriately trained person will choose when to use each situation for wider goals. "Danger" and "opportunity" are said to be dual meanings for the Chinese word "crisis" (Task Force Report 1976), and it is this fundamental principle which distinguishes the PHC opportunistic method from the specialist cohort method. The former builds when the situation is ripe for a change, the latter makes appointments and plans which are not necessarily felt to be opportune when received by the patients or their families. The former starts with a professional discipline in every PHC consultation, the latter can fragment the provision of PHC into specialised sectors.

3) Skills and Practices in Opportunistic Anticipatory Care

Research which has set out to measure people's health-protective behaviours (HPB) in the United States has shown that most people in a sample of 842 respondents practised between 5 and 19 HPBs (mean = 12 and median = 11). In other words, Americans will express a very broad range of behaviours which they consider protect their health. For example, when asked to describe "the three most important things you do to protect your health" (Harris and Guten 1979):

71% mentioned nutrition, foods, eating conditions, etc.
46%   sleep, rest, relaxation
35%   exercise
18%   contact with the health system
14%   personal hygiene
12%   psychological, mental and emotional well-being
 9%   watching weight
 8%   limiting/avoiding tobacco
 7%   medication
 4%   alcohol

The top three all concern everyday personal choices/habits, whereas only about one in five mentioned compliance or contact with professionals; hence the majority had very positive and personal concepts which were confirmed by an analysis of behaviours which gave the following priority order:

66% diet
66% sleep
65% emergency telephone numbers
56% relaxation
53% first-aid kit
52% destroy old medicines

51% check up
47% prayer/religious discipline
47% weight awareness
46% exercise

When Welsh mothers were asked what they do to keep their families healthy, diet/nutrition ranked top of the list (Pill and Stott 1982), but the range of health behaviours they mentioned spontaneously in response to the open-ended question was much more limited than in the American study and there was a strong tendency for the young working-class Welsh mothers to take health for granted, with less personal responsibility for its maintenance. Less than half of a sample of Middlesbrough mothers (UK) thought that heart disease was preventable, but they, too, placed nutrition, stress and exercise at the top of their list of important factors (Cleveland Health Education Department 1982).

The importance of the public's emphasis on the simple life-style factors for health has been well shown by Breslow and Enstrom (1980) in their longitudinal studies in Almeda County, USA. An analysis of many personal and clinical life-style factors showed that seven very basic day-to-day decisions summated to produce a profound impact on life expectancy. The seven factors were:

eating breakfast daily
no snacks between meals
moderate exercise two to three times per day
no cigarette smoking
alcohol in moderation
not overwieght
7–8 hours' sleep per night.

A health score constructed from these seven items had a remarkable assocation with standardised mortality rates (SMRs) (Table 5.2) and these methods are currently being reapplied to a national probability sample of United States citizens by the National Centre for Health Statistics (Schoenborn and Danchik 1980) because of the important implications which arise from this work.

Table 5.2. Health habits and mortality (Breslow and Enstrom 1980)

1965 Health score	Deaths in 9½ years		
	Observed	Expected	SMR
0–3	99	55	178
4–5	388	355	109
6–7	230	305	75

Clinicians need to consider these data very carefully because, when the priorities placed by medical people on life-style are not similar to those of the public, the potential for change is weaker and there is a danger that PHC clinicians and the medical media will lose sight, for example, of the public's felt priority for diet/nutrition at a time when cigarette smoking has become a fashionable focus of attack. Yet malnutrition in its various forms is still a major

69

enemy of most nations and a large number of mothers still lack specific and practical nutritional skills even when they hold a general belief in the importance of food. The single-minded and single-factor approach of many scientists and advertisers to health habits is also at variance with the fairly complex and sometimes ambiguous ideas held by the public.

The research findings have great relevance to the design of health education campaigns and the strategy which PHC personnel can adopt in their work with the public, because in the past the health consumers' views and values have often been ignored by professional educators and clinicians. Furthermore, the importance of simple life-style choices has been wrongly undervalued by the professionals.

Motivation to change a style of life is usually difficult to achieve and wise clinicians will recognise that they have two broadly different ways in which to approach a problem:

(a) the trigger function, and (b) the groundwork function.

In the former the patient already accepts the need for change and it simply takes an experience or someone in authority to trigger the change. Russell, for example, has shown how advice in general practice to stop smoking, a leaflet and an offer of follow-up will result in about 5% of smokers giving up the habit permanently per annum. He points out that this is more effective than any other single method of health education for smoking (Russell et al. 1979). The groundwork function, on the other hand, is a more gradual and sensitive process of edging people with destructive life-styles towards perception of their habits as a problem and acceptance of the need for change. This is less dramatic than the idea of being a "trigger" for change but no less important and very appropriate within the continuing relationships which develop in PHC, particularly as the reasons for a habit or practice are often complex and only slowly identified by the person(s) involved. A worrying cough, a bout of cystitis, a deep vein thrombosis, or recurrent colds, etc. can each be turned into a motivating force for change or the beginnings of a change of life-style when the clinician is willing to consider both the risk factor and patients' priorities. People respond best to the things they want to hear and so deviations from the basic beliefs have to be introduced slowly and sensitively and those changes which are most likely to succeed are those which are consistent with the patients' priorities. The crudity of much advice about life-styles in which some clinicians indulge is far from the ideals of empathetic groundwork within the patient's context. Educationalists, research academics and interested practitioners need to consider and refine appropriate insight and skills to achieve patient motivation because, despite the limitations of present methods, individual (one to one) methods of education for health are more likely to induce behaviour change than group or mass media methods.

Gatherer et al. (1974) reviewed the evidence for the efficacy of health education and found that individual methods induced behaviour change in 91% of the studies reviewed compared with 69% and 67% in group and mass methods respectively, and similar conclusions have come from two reviews of American health education (Task Force Report 1976; Bartlett 1980). However, this does not imply that one-to-one techniques can replace other methods. On the contrary, the reviewers emphasised that the aim should be to encourage all groups in society to consider the importance of life-style in an informed way. Primary health care has a very important role by virtue of the large number of one-to-one contacts with the public, but the media, schools, voluntary organisations and educational institutions also have potential groundwork or trigger functions which remain relatively untapped in most societies.

Skills and Organisation

The skills which can be used to assist in opportunistic motivation of patients in PHC are classifiable into six broad categories.

1) Observation alone.
2) Simple advice.
3) Negotiation.
4) Uses of aids or demonstrations.
5) Involvement of aides/other helpers.
6) Fieldwork and community involvement.

1) In the first category of *observation alone*, the clinician simply notes a risk factor in the patient's life-style: "smokes 20/day" or "obesity" or "very poor diet" or "withdrawing from society" may be entered on the record card even when the issue has not been discussed with the patient. The entry stands as a reminder that this person or family is at risk and the opportunity to explore the matter further or offer help must be taken when the time is ripe.

2) *"Advice"* is commonplace: "You must stop eating so much fat and sugar, Mrs Jones"; "I advise you to give up smoking if you want to enjoy good health in 10 years time"; "Mrs P., your baby will do best on breast"; "For goodness sake, stop taking those damn sleeping tablets, they do you no good" . . . such comments are classified as well-intentioned advice which is occasionally heeded but often ignored when it is one sided and given without adequate cognisance of the factors and pressures which prevent it from being acted upon. However, it is also true that the family physician who knows his patients well can appear to be abrupt and one sided whereas in reality the advice is given within a continuing relationship of understanding and trust which has been earned by years of commitment to the family. Firm advice on one occasion which is a fragment of a continuing negotiation within the doctor–patient relationship is often effective, as Russell et al. (1979) and others have shown, but it is likely that those who work in PHC will find that the maintenance of a trusting relationship will continue to be more important than any media campaign in helping people to discover healthy habits.

3) *Negotiation* is a two-way process in which the doctor and patient (or relative) consider the issues at stake. It is a skill which can only be learned by those who value and hear the other person's viewpoint, not as a history to be recorded but as a set of values, attitudes and pressures which are felt and which can facilitate or stand in the way of change.

Doctor: "It appears that you are having some difficulty with breast-feeding, you seem most unhappy about it."

71

Patient: "Yes doctor, I known that it is good for him but it is so painful."
Doctor: "Painful?" (gentle tone).
Patient: "Every night my husband tells me to mix a bottle for the baby and to stop stretching my breasts with milk . . . he hates me breast-feeding."

The barriers to breast-feeding successfully in this poor woman came to light through a negotiating attitude, and in some sections of society such feelings are common and are unlikely to be overcome unless breast-feeding is managed as a family issue.

The teaching of specific skills (e.g. back exercises, avoidance of home accidents, relaxation methods, food choices, etc.) also requires a negotiating aproach to be sure that the patient can accept the relevance and apply the new skill successfully as unexpected barriers can prevent the implementation of quite simple techniques. Skilled interviewing (see Chap. 1) is an essential prelude to skilled negotiations with patients, as is some understanding of the antecedents of health behaviours.

4) *Use of aids*, posters, pamphlets, instruction booklets, diagrams, even slides or videotape, which are available from many sources, will help the PHC clinician reinforce messages. These are important adjuncts to the verbal skills of categories (2) and (3), but the clinician must be aware that people's interpretations of the same scene can vary greatly. Some tribal Africans have difficulty in interpreting three-dimensional pictures and many highly intelligent people looking at the same poster will express quite different emphases. For example, Leathar (1980) has shown how commercial advertising does more than simply project a brand name or point out how good a product is in technical terms. Often it tries to surround the objective message by warm and attractive feelings which contain elements of trust, honesty, sympathy or style. In short, it creates feelings of "that's for me". Leathar found that it was very difficult to make people pay continued attention to heavily negative visual material. For example, a poster which presented a cigarette as a tombstone in a graveyard was perceived by nonsmokers as an antismoking message, but smokers were very likely to see the cigarette as an unrelated object such as a stick of rock or lipstick or a telegraph pole.

Psychological defences and denial introduce powerful distortions to people's perceptions of pictures and so many aids (pamphlets, posters, etc.) when used in isolation are of limited value, whereas those that are clear and simple, if used to illustrate or stimulate discussion, can have a powerful effect when the timing is opportune and the discussant is respected and trusted. Aids which facilitate discussion are helpful but aids which are pushed across the table to replace negotiation are likely to be misunderstood. Research is urgently needed to assess the design of simple aids for effective use in the PHC context because ordinary advertising techniques are often inappropriate. Pencil-and-paper diagrams drawn during discussion with a trusted clinician may prove to be hard to beat as they combine personal with factual elements.

5) Involvement of aides and others. ⎱
⎰ To be considered together.
6) Fieldwork and community participation. ⎰

Those who develop the skill to clairify people's beliefs, motivation and barriers to a possible change of life-style soon come to realise that the process of health behaviour change is complex and difficult for most people. The medical view on smoking, drinking, eating habits, sexuality, drug usage, home organisation, relationships, relaxation and recreation is a minor consideration in most people's decisions, and the probability for change is small if the medical view is not reasonably concordant with the realities of personal conviction and the pressures from family, social and work environments (see Fig. 5.1).

John (38 years) laughed inwardly when his doctor suggested that he should reduce his tobacco consumption . . . his wife, father, mother and friends all smoked as they chatted, drank and worked together . . . life would be a mockery without the tobacco he loved and the thought of sitting in his smoke-filled parlour without a cigarette in his hand was to him a bizarre idea.

The process of change in a society which is quite fixed in its ways is unlikely to be speeded more than minimally by clinical exhortation unless some of the pressures and barriers which impede change from destructive life-styles can be modified; thus the clinician who tries to provoke/encourage change often has to choose to do so only when the change is most likely or explore the barriers to change instead. Two important perspectives have been pointed out in this regard. First, that small changes in a community can have ripple effects and lead to other changes. Hence, a small response in individuals can become a significant response in the community over a period of years as each individual influences others. Work with smokers (Russell et al. 1979) and malnourished children (Stott 1976) has been shown to fulfil this principle and many educators have further anecdotal support for it. The "ripple effect" is most likely if patients receive reinforcement which is practical and relevant to their problem.

A second perspective is that the opportunistic method in PHC will only yield definite results if community participation is invoked. Tones (1979) emphasised the community participation approach in his review and he quoted projects of this type which tripled attendances for cervical cytology, improved nutritional knowledge, decreased truancy, enhanced educational achievements, increased home ownership, lowered prevalence of upper respiratory infections and reduced chronic otitis media in different communities. Community participation and the use of aides who bridge the gap between professional PHC and the community are two well-researched methods which are little used in developed countries, yet increasingly applied in the less privileged parts of the world. Both are important components of the repertoire of organisational skills which should be available to those who work in PHC.

Many PHC clinicians never progress conceptually beyond category (2) or category (3) in the six-fold classification of skills for opportunistic anticipatory care and it is not the purpose of this text to discuss why this should be. However, every student should be capable of classifying opportunistic anticipatory care into six approaches for every clinical risk factor/problem, and examples of these classifications have been included in Tables 5.3–5.6 for smoking, tension, malnutrition and home accidents to illustrate a simple yet practical hierarchy of skills and organisation. Students of PHC should also be capable of describing the many factors which contribute to health behaviour (see Fig. 5.1) which is so patently multidimensional (Williams and Wechsler 1972; Langlie 1977) and subject to many very effective barriers.

Table 5.3. Six approaches to smoking problem

Need	Methods available	Examples of opening comments and techniques
Smoking habit*	1) State nature of problem	"Smoking is damaging your lungs/heart etc."
	2) An instruction/specific recommendation	"It is essential that you stop smoking and I suggest you do it in this way . . ."
	3) Negotiating method to explore barriers, beliefs and motivation	"People smoke for many different reasons" or "I wonder whether you have ever considered giving up smoking?"
	4) Use of aids to extend (2) or (3)	Information leaflets/programmes to help identify reasons for smoking Behaviour-modification programmes Audiovisual aids Smoking substitutes
	5) Involve aides to extend (2) or (3)	Smoking clinic Psychologist Psychotherapy Hypnosis Acupuncture
	6) Fieldwork and/or community involvement, to reinforce needs/skills and modify barriers	Involvement of family Involvement of social group Campaign locally

*The interested reader is referred to Emery et al. (1968) and Russell et al. (1979).

Table 5.4. Six approaches to management of nonspecific tension

Need	Method available	Examples of opening comments and techniques
Tension*	1) Define nature of problem	"Tension is at the root of your problem."
	2) An instruction/specific recommendation	"It is essential that you find more time to relax. I suggest . . ."
	3) Negotiating methods to explore barriers, beliefs and motivation	"I suspect you feel that tension contributes to your problems"
		or
		"You seem to be feeling very tense — do you think that this can be overcome?"
	4) Use of aids to extend (2) or (3)	Information sheets
		Programmes to help the individual relax (e.g. audio-cassette for home use)
		Audiovisual aids
		Short-term tranquillisers
		Relaxation skills teaching
	5) Involve aides to extend (2) or (3)	Psychologist
		Acupuncture
		Hypnosis
		Therapists of various types
	6) Fieldwork and/or community involvement which reinforce needs/skills and modify barriers	Family involvement/therapy
		Social group involvement
		Attempts to modify environment if it is a cause of stress

*The interested reader will recognise a vast literature on this subject and the truism that most tension is physiological with definite, albeit multifactorial, causes which need to be identified.

Table 5.5. Six approaches to prevention of malnutrition

Need	Methods available	Examples of opening comments and techniques
A change of diet due to malnutrition (obesity or undernutrition)*	1) To state the nature of the problem	"Your child is very underweight."
	2) An instruction or specific recommendation	"Your child will not grow normally unless he has more of x, y and z."
	3) Negotiating method to attempt to identify the barriers, beliefs and motivations	"I wonder if you are happy about your family's diet?"
	4) Use of aids to extend (2) or (3)	Diet sheets Booklets Visual displays Audiovisual aids
	5) Involve aides to extend (2) or (3)	Dietician } Nutrition demonstrator } Choice, preparation and presentation of foods Health visitor Social worker
	6) Fieldwork and/or community involvement to reinforce needs/skills and help modify barriers to change	Home visiting by aide/doctor/nurse Key figures/groups in community Availability of foods Production of foods Political considerations

*The interested reader is referred to the text to avoid simplistic interpretation of the causes of malnutrition.

Table 5.6. Six approaches to prevention of home accidents

Need	Method available	Examples of opening comments and techniques
Home accidents*	1) State nature of problem	"That fire/stove/cupboard, it is very dangerous."
	2) Specific recommendation	"You really must get a guard for that fire/stove . . . . I suggest you go and see . . ."
	3) Negotiating method to explore barriers, beliefs and motivation	"Accidents in the home cause us more and more concern . . . have you considered whether there are risks you could modify?"
	4) Use of aids to extend (2) or (3)	Information sheets
		Visual aids
		Audiovisual programmes
	5) Involve aides to extend (2) or (3)	Health visitors
		Teachers
		District nurses
		Social workers
	6) Fieldwork and/or community involvement which reinforces needs/skills and modifies barriers	Family involvement at home
		Police
		Fire officers ⎱ Individual and group work
		Ambulance men ⎰
		Housing Dept. ⎱ Political pressure
		Parks Dept. ⎰

*The interested reader is referred to the section on accidents and destructive behaviours to gain a more comprehensive understanding of the reasons for accidents.

77

4) Priorities for Anticipatory Care

The establishment of priorities for anticipatory care is a task for individual areas in the light of local needs and facilities, but two broadly different sets of opportunities exist in all areas.

1) Disorder-specific opportunities.
2) Nonspecific opportunities.

The first group includes all those conditions for which procedures are available to prevent/anticipate specific problems and in which clinical intervention is likely to be beneficial (e.g. immunisation). The second group includes life-style and other factors which have an impact on a wide range of possible disorders and are thus nonspecific but broadly based in their effects. For example, diet and smoking both have an impact on a very large number of diseases. A listing produced by the Royal College of General Practitioners (1981) failed to separate these two groups, so here the RCGP list has been revised and abbreviated to demonstrate the important division (Table 5.7). Many of the items on the left side of the table are similar to the Breslow and Enstrom (1980) factors described earlier (see page 69), whereas most of those on the right-hand column involve clinical procedures and therefore qualify easily as conventional medical tasks.

Table 5.7. Examples of specific and nonspecific opportunities for anticipatory care

Nonspecific opportunities	Specific opportunities
Breast-feeding	Family planning
Diet choices	Immunisation
Hygiene	Neural tube defects
Smoking	Phenylketonuria
Alcohol excess	Squint and visual problems
Drug excesses	Congenital dislocation of hip
Exercise	Dental caries '
Rest and recreation	Hearing problems
Relationships (including spiritual)	Hypothyroidism
Accident prevention	Male descent of testes
	Venereal disease
	Hypertension in young adults
	Cancer of bladder
	Cancer of cervix
	Cancer of skin
	Pulmonary tuberculosis
	Urinary infection in pregnancy

One curious muddle which has crept into some doctors' thinking is to consider most clinical tasks as being preventive in nature: primary (as in immunisation), secondary (as in early disease detection) and tertiary (when complications of established disease are prevented). This nomenclature is, in the author's view, unhelpful because it lulls the curative-minded clinician into believing that preventive medicine is practised every time a prescription is signed, a screening test is done, an injection given or an operation performed. "Preventive care", said the Working Party on Healthier Children, "conveys the idea of doctors constantly keeping prevention in mind" (Royal College of General Practitioners 1982). A laudable sentiment this may be, but clinicians who are steeped in curative traditions need no encouragement to go on practising curative medicine under the new name of prevention. Primary prevention is totally different from so-called secondary or tertiary prevention. Furthermore, to pretend that the nonspecific cluster of opportunities with a broad impact on health (Table 5.7) lies on a continuum with the clinically specific screening procedures is to be blind to an international trend and reorientation of responsibilities, skills and attitudes which faces the medical profession and society. We cannot eschew some responsibility for encouraging people to adopt the nonspecific group of opportunities without raising serious ethical questions about professionalism in PHC, an issue which is returned to later.

A second common confusion lies between health education and disease education (Task Force Report 1976), authors often speaking of the former when they mean the latter, particularly in relation to chronic disease. This confusion devalues the importance of education for true prevention and can lull clinicians into thinking that appropriate sharing of information about chronic diseases is somehow comparable in impact on the community to the prevention of a range of potential disorders by modification of simple risk factors. In terms of the framework (see Fig. 2.1), all disease education belongs to current and continuing problems (Areas A and C) and, important as disease education is, it is a rather watered-down form of prevention.

Enthusiasts who have pioneered specific aspects of anticipatory care in PHC do, however, deserve special mention because they have highlighted many developments: Curtis Jenkins (1980) and his work on paediatric development surveillance, Tudor Hart (1980) in his contribution to hypertension screening and management, Marsh and Kaim-Caudle (1976) in the integration of nursing, social and lay workers in Western PHC, and Stott (senior) (1976) in his application of the "referral chain" approach to malnutrition management and prevention in a Zulu community. Each of these men has pioneered methods and skills to develop his field of special concern and each has modified a primary care base to accept anticipatory PHC innovations, either because circumstances demanded a priority and/or because his individual special interests determined the priority. Others in PHC who are not so single minded may be less motivated to focus on a special theme, but the impact of their PHC professional involvement will nevertheless depend on both the depth and the breadth of their approaches to anticipatory care and its relevance to local community needs. Generalists would be wise if they look carefully at the results of the pioneers of new principles and methods. Others, when describing priorities for anticipatory PHC, have usually emphasised activities with a large clinical procedural element. Immunisation, contraception and antenatal (fetal) care are often near the top of the lists in official reports (Consultative Document 1976; Royal College of General Practitioners 1981, 1982), and so important growth points in anticipatory PHC will be illustrated by considering three examples which have received less attention.

1) Nutrition.
2) Prevention of destructive behaviour.
3) Developmental scanning.

The reader will notice that two of the three are more concerned with behaviour than clinical procedures and the third is a fair mixture of both.

1) *Nutrition* has been described as "the cornerstone of prevention, the handmaiden of curative medicine and the responsibility of every physician" (Journal of Clinical Nutrition 1953) because it is the most basic of all our material needs; yet, paradoxically, nutrition receives very little attention from a high proportion of practising clinicians who seem to have been lulled into accepting overnutrition and its sequelae as an inevitable consequence of an affluent life-style, and various grades of undernutrition as the inevitable results of poverty. To answer that the undernourished are to blame for their plight and the overnourished have chosen to be fat by their greedy habits is a cruel oversimplification, because famine is often the product of politics or ignorance and appetite can no longer be regarded as a reliable guide to our nutritional needs. The art and science of food technology have so transformed the appearance, taste and content of many natural foodstuffs that appetite is a poor guide to health and the public needs assistance with its choices (Pearce and Crocker 1944; Hume Hall 1974; British Nutrition Foundation 1975; Yellowlees 1979) – "the great taste-bud deceit".

Many modern food modifications could be used to illustrate the great taste-bud deceit, but an obvious example of food transformation with unfortunate results is the reduction in fibre content which pleases the public's palate and contributes to its diseases. It is indicative of our age that both fibre depletion and fibre enrichment have been exploited commercially, and some doctors continue to lose valuable opportunities for encouraging sound diet modification by prescribing fibre in medicinal form instead of encouraging the person concerned to consider dietary changes to achieve the same objective more sensibly.

> *Patient:* "But doctor I have taken laxatives on and off since my baby was born 3 years ago . . . can't I have a new bottle of x?"
> *Doctor:* "Mrs P., you have been thrashing your tired bowel with laxatives for all these years . . . I'm suggesting that it can be helped to become fit and active once more if you give it some roughage to work on."
> *Patient:* "What does that entail doctor?"

Clinical staff in PHC have numerous opportunities to encourage sensible decisions about the substances people choose to send down their oro-gastrointestinal tracts, and sound eating habits have an impact on many different aspects of health: periodontal disease, dental decay, dyspepsia, constipation, diverticular disease, irritable bowel, diabetes mellitus, obesity, malnutrition syndromes, some congenital anomalies, ischaemic heart disease, cerebral function, hypertension, certain malignancies and many other conditions have faulty nutrition among their antecedent factors (Passmore et al. 1979).

Prophets of despair often cite diet as too complex a subject for the public to cope with, but there is overwhelming evidence that a healthy adult diet should be varied and rich in fresh foods (fruit, vegetables and salads) and unprocessed foods, but not dominated by foods with a high fat or salt content (US Senate Select Committee on Nutrition and Human Needs 1978; Passmore et al. 1979). The United States Department of Health, Education and Welfare, in conjunction with the Department of Agriculture, has issued dietary guidelines for the American people (Table 5.8) which are simple enough to be grasped by most people yet compatible with the more detailed and complex Select Committee Report on Nutrition and Human Needs which was published by the US Senate in 1978 (Tables 5.9 and 5.10). The guidelines in Table 5.8 are also in broad agreement with recommendations from other countries (British Nutrition Foundation 1975; US Senate Select Committee on Nutrition and Human Needs 1978; Passmore et al. 1979).

Table 5.8. Dietary guidelines (US Departments of Agriculture and Health Education and Welfare 1980)

Eat a variety of food
Maintain an ideal weight
Avoid too much fat, saturated fat and cholesterol
Eat foods with adequate starch and fibre
Avoid too much sugar
Avoid too much sodium
If you drink alcohol, do so in moderation

Table 5.9. "Dietary goals for USA" (US Senate Select Committee 1978)

1) To avoid being over weight
2) To increase consumption of complex carbohydrates and naturally occurring sugars from about 28% to about 48% of energy intake; and to reduce the consumption of refined and processed sugars by about 45% to account for about 10% of total energy intake
3) Reduce overall fat consumption from approximately 40% to approximately 30% of energy intake
4) Reduce saturated fat consumption to account for about 10% of total energy intake
5) Reduce cholesterol consumption to about 300 g/day
6) Limit sodium intake by reducing salt intake to about 5 g/day

Table 5.10. Ways in which to accomplish dietary goals for USA (shown in Table 5.9)

1) Increased consumption of fats, vegetables and whole grain
2) Decreased consumption of refined and processed sugars and foods high in such sugars
3) Decreased consumption of food high in total fat and particularly to replace saturated fats, whether obtained from animal or vegetable sources, with polyunsaturated fats
4) Decreased consumption of animal fat and choice of meat, poultry and fish that will reduce saturated fat intake
5) Except for young children, substitute low-fat dairy products for high-fat dairy products

The recommended changes in national diets are largely away from energy-dense foods (usually those with high energy but low volume). It is therefore vital to point out that what is good for adults or older children is not necessarily right for younger children and infants who are normally reared on a most remarkable substance – milk – which is a liquid with a very high energy density by virtue of its content of emulsified fats. Young children are physically unable to consume the solid energy-dense foods enjoyed by adults and there is growing evidence that watery gruels/soups which often form the basis of weaning diets in poor communities provide so little energy per unit volume that children have to consume huge quantities of the liquid or semisolid mixtures to get the calories they need to grow (Church 1979); their pot-bellies provide a physical indicator of the volume they have to imbibe (assuming other causes of abdominal distension are excluded). Myths about theoretical protein needs have been well challenged by Mclaren (1975) who showed how large-scale nutrition intervention campaigns based on theoretical requirements can have an adverse effect on malnutrition by placing too much emphasis on new concentrated protein foods instead of building on traditional dietary patterns and practices.

The importance of nutrient density and viscosity in human nutrition was highlighted by Church, whose diagrams are presented in Table 5.11 and Figs. 5.3 and 5.4.

Table 5.11. Feeding and stages of development (Church 1979)

Stage	Fetal	Birth	Infant phase (6–12 months)	Toddler phase (2 years)
Appropriate form of food and water	Intravenous	Liquid	Semisolid gruel or pap	Mixed family foods
Means of feeding	Placenta	Breast- or bottle-feeding	Feeding by mother, by hand or utensil	Self-feeding
Child skills	None	Ability to suck and swallow	Development of chewing	Co-ordination of hand–mouth feeding skills
Psychological stages	Confluence and passivity	Dependence on mother	Decreasing dependency	Growth of independence, identity
Developmental stages	Weaning from the womb	"In arms" phase	Crawling phase	Walking

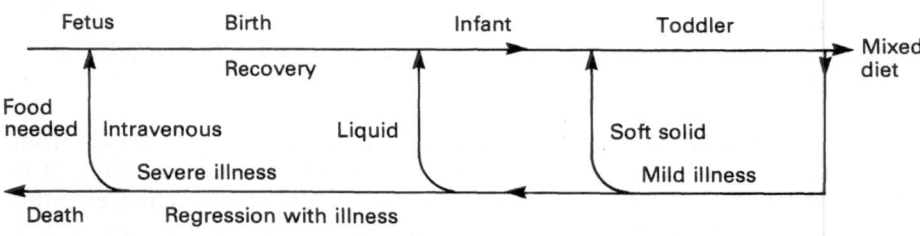

Fig. 5.3. A schematic diagram of the effect of illness on feeding (Church 1979).

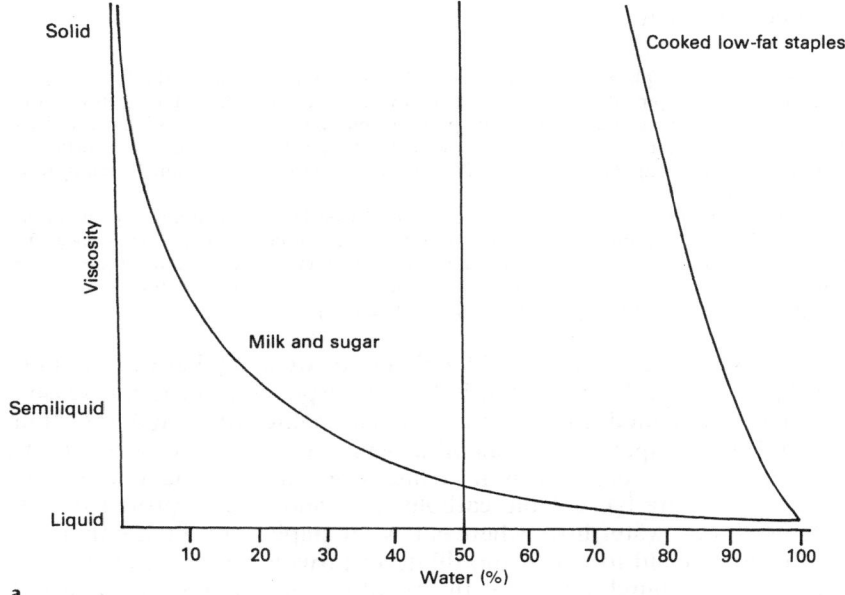

a

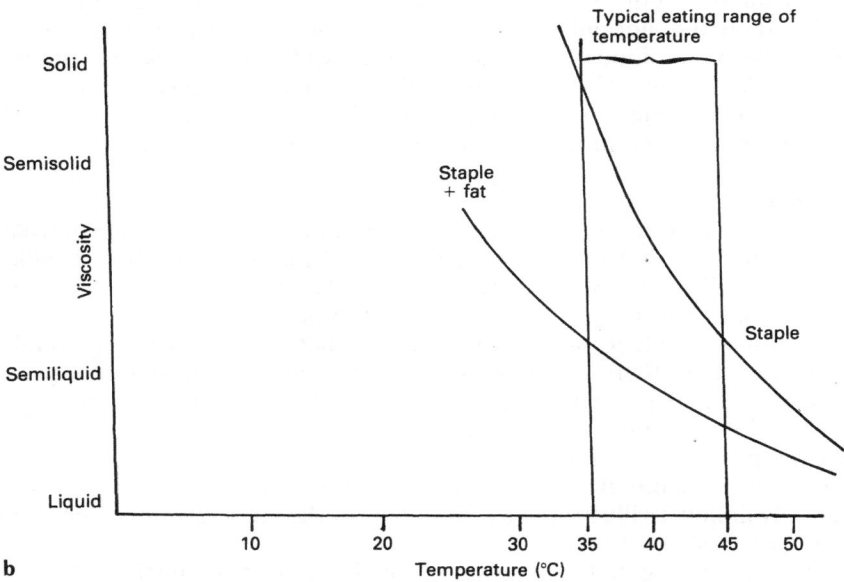

b

Fig. 5.4. Factors affecting the viscosity of food. **a** The viscosity of cooked foods is most basically affected by dilution with water, but varies enormously with different ingredients and with temperature. The most important factors are solubility of the ingredients and the amount of fat. The range of variability is illustrated by the curves for milk and cooked staples. **b** All foods become thicker with cooling, but the addition of fat dramatically reduces the rate of change (Church 1979).

Church points out that:

> Food viscosity is, from a physiological and developmental point of view, a vital factor . . . at various phases of development only food of the right viscosity can be adequately dealt with (as shown in Table 5.11). Some of the features are primarily physiological and neurological, such as the ability to suck, chew or swallow, whereas others relate to skills such as eating or drinking which are vital for the young child who has to fight for its own share from a communal family dish (poorer communities).
>
> Adequate weaning from milk to solid mixed diet is obviously fundamentally dependent on foods of suitable viscosity. Illness has a regressive effect, which is clinically well recognised and illustrated (Fig. 5.3). The more severe the illness, the further the regression, requiring the appropriate means of feeding to be modified back towards the intravenous route. Recovery involves passing rapidly through the normal developmental phases.

It is clear from the data that a child with a poor weaning diet will run into nutritional problems each time that he is ill. This is a possible nutritional reason for the well-documented association between malnutrition and infection (Scrimshaw 1964). Important factors influencing the viscosity of food are its water content, its temperature, its fat content and its ingredient solubility, hence milk containing fat, soluble carbohydrate and soluble protein is still drinkable at 200 ml water/litre, whereas low-fat staples are often either too thick or dry for a child to eat or too dilute to provide sufficient energy for childhood growth. Church illustrates this point by showing how a 1-year-old child on a typical maize gruel in central Africa would need 4 litres of food whereas an older sibling eating the same meals in a more solid form would consume a quarter of the volume for the same energy content. The addition of fat to the staple diet not only adds energy by virtue of its density (38 kJ or 9 kcal/g), it also makes food more palatable over a wider range of water content (Fig. 5.4). Workers in well-fed nations will, of course, recognise the opposite danger, namely a surplus of high energy-dense foods due to artificial emulsification and concentrated tinned semisolids too early in life.

To summarise:

a) Nutrition is relevant to every sphere of PHC and the basic concepts of what represents the best diet for adults (see Table 5.8) and infants (breast-milk) (Jelliffe and Jelliffe 1975) is not too complicated for grass-roots workers. Indeed, we dare not make it too complicated to be useful.

b) Scientific knowledge about nutrition and dietetics is expanding rapidly and as this happens there is a progressive re-awakening of the need for great caution when food is modified by technological processes which increase energy density or add foreign chemicals. The dilution of adult foods does not necessarily produce an infant food.

c) Poverty and ignorance may co-exist as factors in malnutrition but they are not causally linked, as illustrated by the impact of the great taste-bud deceit on affluent societies.

d) Those practising PHC can only give a higher priority to nutritional issues in their areas by asking themselves and others "Who helps/teaches people to choose/produce food more wisely and to protect its nutrient content during preparation for eating?"

e) The social context in which food is grown, purchased, prepared and served has to be taken into account if nutritional advice is to be relevant and practical for the individual family. This leads to the inevitable conclusion that centralised recommendations can only be useful if they are negotiated at the local level by people who are trained to take specialist advice and modify it in primary health care to make it compatible with the needs of local communities.

2) Accidents and *destructive behaviours* are often regarded as results of a social fabric which can enmesh the individual and make a personal change very difficult. Family therapists (Kingston 1982), sociologists (Langlie 1977) and many doctors often feel that the individual is unlikely to change habits unless the social network changes. Of course, environmental factors which inhibit personal changes have also been incriminated as determinants of accidents and destructive behaviours. Blaxter (1981) conducted an extensive study of cycles of deprivation in Aberdeen and concluded that the major influences on ill-health of children were still air pollution and economic disadvantage, with remedies to be found in environmental policies, traffic control and housing design rather than the behaviour of individual families. Similar conclusions have been reached by students of the poverty trap in less developed areas and developed nations (Black 1980; Stacey 1980).

The PHC doctor/nurse/health visitor/aide is often in the difficult position of observing hazards to children or adults in the home or local environment and wondering what, if anything, to do or say. Open fires, unguarded stoves, chemicals, unlocked medicines, dangerous stairs, slippery floor coverings, poor ventilation, dangerous heaters, unguarded pits or ponds, hazardous windows, destructive relationships, poor food storage, bad habits, filthy home environments, chaotic electrical fittings and many other hazards confront those who keep their eyes and ears open on their clinical rounds. Are these all opportunities for tactful enquiry or comment or does that convert the professional into a policeman? Is offering help with a drinking, smoking, dietetic or drug problem interference or caring? The answers to these questions are not always straightforward because the professional can be torn between wanting to offer advice/help and feeling that it is unlikely to be taken in a poor environment with poor motivation or when chronically ill inhabitants are involved. One unsatisfactory solution to this dilemma is to ignore the problems and deal with "medical" issues only:

Nurse P. stumbled over broken glass as she walked up the garden path to the grubby front door. The garden was littered with rubbish and she winced at the smell of unswept rooms inhabited by cats and dogs as the front door opened. The old man's leg ulcers were dressed quickly, but she had to push away a dog who was determined to lick his master's raw flesh; then she retreated, gasping for fresh air as she left the house. On the table she passed an unnoticed and unopened pile of full medicine bottles. She stopped at the gate and scribbled a report for the nursing officer: "Mr J. leg ulcers dressed with Eusol."

Psychological shut-off makes impossible tasks tolerable and most young doctors or nurses who have worked at the sharp end of community care must be well aware of having fled from some disgusting or horrible scenes in ghastly homes where the apparently intractable problems inhibit the exercise of compassionate logic or numb any determination to change a society which can allow or encourage such squalor. A quick prescription or a wound dressing can permit a professionally acceptable departure, but it leaves the situation unchanged.

"Risk mindedness" is both a skill and a discipline because every person/family is subject to different modifiable risk and only those with local knowledge of important hazards to health are likely to identify opportunities for changes in the environment, home or personal habits. There is evidence that personal, specific and practical help/advice about hazards in the home is more effective than media campaigns (Gatherer et al. 1974; Colver et al. 1982), particularly if the helper has a respected professional role. In areas where good hygiene or affluence is prominent, the danger of overlooking risks to the family health and safety still exists and it is unthinkable that a caring PHC professional could "pass by" obvious hazards because of a theory that people are trapped in life-style patterns. Yet there is another trap: treating the results of disordered lives and environments can dominate the PHC so much and prove so emotionally draining that there can be insufficient time for thoughts of prevention. This is a vicious circle which modern PHC must break into.

In the nineteenth century, great physicians used their influence to bring changes to the whole of society. Dr Southwood Smith, who condemned the squalor of his patients' environments, was the person who primed the social reformers of the day. He invoked the support of Chadwick, Shaftesbury and Bentham, who arose with political support, and he enlisted the help of an artist and an author (Charles Dickens) to highlight the poverty in his patients' lives which caused such ill-health. William Farr, the first Registrar General of England and Wales, left his practice to produce the early health statistics, and the great Rudolf Virchow left cellular pathology to campaign for sewage disposal and hygiene in German public places. All these great men used their knowledge, their experiences and their status to influence public reform in health matters. They all primed the reformers and demanded a change from purely curative attitudes.

Who, we must ask, are the latter-day Smiths, Farrs and Virchows? If great strides in public health were stimulated by clinicians, who could see the problems and the opportunities for prevention, what should clinicians be doing today to tackle the huge problems of accidents in or near the home, smoking, drinking excesses, drug abuse, social withdrawal and antisocial acts?

Two types of action are clearly visible on the available evidence.

a) Political action to improve housing, inner-city play areas for children, opportunities for recreation and exercise, safety at work and economic hardship, etc.
b) Personal action against choices of life-style which are leading to ill-health and an environment which encourages the next generation to have equally poor habits.

Professionals in PHC have the status and skill to act collectively as a pressure group to get improvements with relevant authorities – as they have done to influence smoking and clean air in some countries. They are also in privileged and responsible positions individually which can be used to influence patients' decisions about personal risk taking. The marriage of collective and personal responsibility for health is a marker of the new era in public health, an era which recognises that both central and peripheral actions are essential if accidental and behavioural causes of illness and death are to be diminished in the future.

"Risk mindedness" will eventually become entrenched as a skill and a discipline for all PHC workers, but each will have to learn to guard against being numbed by seemingly impossible odds when poverty is rife, or being conveniently blind when affluent life-styles embrace destructive habits or attitudes.

3) *Developmental scanning.* Objective measurements have transformed the developmental assessment of children from being an impressionistic exercise into the beginning of a science, and major reports have now argued strongly for systematic surveillance of all healthy children (Department of Health and Social Security 1976; Royal College of General Practitioners 1982), despite the fact that many of the methods used do not stand up to the scrutiny that Wilson (1965) (Table 5.12) or Cochrane and Holland (1971) proposed for all screening procedures. The debate about the effectiveness of various screening

Table 5.12. Criteria to judge whether a screening test is justified. (After Wilson 1965)

The condition should be important
An accepted treatment must be available for the condition
The facilities for diagnosis and treatment must be available
A latent or early symptomatic stage must exist
A sensitive and specific screening test must be available
The test must be acceptable to the population
The natural history of the condition must be understood
An agreed treatment policy must exist
The cost must be acceptable
Case finding must be a continuing process

procedures in children will probably continue for a long time (Royal College of General Practitioners 1982), but the reality in international terms is that detailed childhood developmental assessment is likely to remain a luxury for the few. Indeed, developmental paediatricians will have done the public a grave disservice if specialised developmental assessment distracts general clinicians to being more technical than commonsensical in their dealings with children. Tape measures, linear scales and percentile charts are vital to the training of the competent clinician while gathering experience, but are they relevant to most PHC fieldwork? Just as classical clinical history taking becomes truncated and more focused with experience, so formal developmental assessment needs to be condensed into a "developmental scan" on every child seen in PCH. Here, speed and relevance are more important than detailed comprehensive coverage of every detail, and being constantly alert is more appropriate than occasional special screening exercises.

The great strength of PHC is that children with developmental delay usually have an above-average number of problems with behaviour, social circumstances or recurrent infections (Bax et al. 1980) and so they come to PHC services anyway (Zinken and Cox 1976). Most opportunities for developmental scanning present for other reasons (Sackett and Holland 1975; Morrell 1978) and much of this potential may be lost if clinicians are encouraged to pigeon-hole their developmental thinking to a "speical clinic once a week" or "leave it to the specialist". "One clinic per activity" is the ideal of the super-specialist, but the generalist who tries to work in this way is courting organisational disaster and massive inconvenience for patients because special clinics can proliferate and their value is far from proven in PHC, despite the enthusiasm of the pioneers who are often more specialist minded than their colleagues.

The need for the generalist to have a broad view of each patient was well made by S.R. Meadows (1977) when he described a candidate for a higher paediatric examination who, when presented with a wizened, malnourished and sad little baby, spent the first 5 minutes of the viva giving an excellent account of the infant's neurological reflexes and visual development but failed to comment on the gross signs which had made the child's general practitioner alarmed. Meadows quite reasonably asked the rhetorical question: "What kind of doctor in PHC would you take your child to?"

A quick and useful developmental scan can only be performed by those who have learned to appreciate the normal patterns of childhood development and the wide range of normality. Only then will danger signals be recognised quickly. For example, the absence of a social smile by 8 weeks, no two-word phrases by 2 years and no three-word sentences by 3 years are regarded as important limits in language development. The balanced cephalocaudal unfolding of extensor flexor locomotor development is also a logical sequence of progress to give good head control by 4–6 months, sitting control by 6–8 months and the vital finger/thumb opposition by 9 months to allow fine manipulation skills to develop. Early awareness of responses to sound and vision is particularly significant because acquired disorders as well as congenital anomalies are at stake. Gross weight and size are also quite narrowly correlated with age in early life and social behaviour is important at all ages.

In PHC, the developmental scan involves making a guestimate of every child's age and stage of development before looking at the recorded date of birth, a discipline which adds virtually nothing to the consultation time because it is largely part of that sound Oslerian tradition of observing carefully and systematically both child and mother–child interaction. Experienced clinicians who have disciplined themselves to learn to "scan" are unlikely to miss important deviations from normal after the neonatal phase, but there is an urgent need for this quick and regular routine in day-to-day PHC to be compared with a battery of occasional developmental tests for effectiveness and efficiency.

Specialised screening at intervals is only logical where regular generalised scanning is ineffective or absent. However, the wide gulf which exists between increasingly detailed developmental paediatrics and those parts of PHC where children are never scanned with developmentally attuned eyes, can be bridged in two ways. Either the specialists extrapolate their detailed techniques to the community, as was suggested in certain reports (Department of Health and Social Security 1976; Royal College of General Practitioners 1982), or the generalists aim to scan all children they see. The former represents specialisation and fragmentation of PHC, the latter the maintenance of a generalised tradition. The most practical and cost-effective method remains to be proven and the onus is now on generalists to prove the value of developmental scanning which is, after all, exactly what many experienced nurses, health visitors and practitioners already do.

Presymptomatic Diagnosis

Presymptomatic diagnosis (screening) is a veritable Pandora's box of opportunities for the PHC clinician, but a box filled with enthusiasm rather than logic, and it is salutory to recall that quite strict criteria have been recommended to test whether a screening procedure is justified (Table 5.12).

Cochrane and Holland (1971), applying criteria similar to those in Table 5.12, decided that, in pre-school children, only the following conditions qualified for screening.

Congenital dislocation of hip.
Phenylketonuria.
Hearing.
Vision.

Rose (1971) applied the same criteria to 14 chronic conditions and found that only five fulfilled the requirements.

Phenylketonuria.
Pulmonary tuberculosis in high-risk groups.
Urinary infections in pregnancy.
Hypertension in young/middle-aged groups.
Chorion carcinoma following hydatidiform mole.

By 1980, the situation had only changed to include glaucoma in the first degree, relatives of sufferers and cervical cytology in high-risk groups; so the clinician can see that the practice of presymptomatic screening vastly exceeds what is scientifically justified, particularly in the fields of developmental paediatrics and routine medical check-ups on otherwise healthy men and women. It is, however, extremely important to differentiate clinical surveillance of patients who have come to PHC for other problems from formal screening of successive cohorts, and here the reader is referred back to the introduction to this chapter in which the opportunism in PHC was compared with screening. Opportunistic surveillance can be conducted for less than definite deviations from normal and these can be monitored unobtrusively and inexpensively by alert and well-organised PHC with or without full patient participation.

Conclusions

The opportunistic integration of health promotion and disease prevention (anticipatory care) into PHC clinical practice requires that clinicians ask themselves whether it is appropriate to try to help each patient to consider the long-term implications of personal life-style and whether a selected screening examination, test or procedure is justified in the interests of future health. The answers to these questions will often be "no" because of the nature of the current problems or restraints, but sometimes it will be "yes" and a relatively minor presenting problem can then become the key to events which may modify future morbidity and life expectancy of the individual or the family. Where primary health care offers a reasonable level of accessibility, availability and continuity, the principle of opportunism appears to be a very effective, efficient and professional method of health promotion provided the skills used are commensurate with the opportunities for their practice.

Success with the principle of opportunism will depend on the insight, skills, timing and priorities of the doctor/nurse/aide and the willingness of the patient/family to participate in a proposed change of habits or use of services. A hierarchy of skills and methods is available for professional workers but the level achieved will depend on the qualities of individual teams and their success at delegation. Detailed priorities for anticipatory care will differ from area to area, but distressing international gradients for morbidity and mortality are unlikely to be reduced until all who are involved in PHC begin to work for the priorities of social justice, reduction of environmental hazards, and sound nutrition. Sometimes, these priorities will demand political action, but often the clinician will be in a position to encourage grass-roots responsibility and actions in a way which will benefit the individual and, by ripple effect, society at large.

Primary health care which is accessible, available and acceptable to the peoples of the world (Stephen 1981) is still an almost untapped resource which, by virtue of its close contact with the populace, should wield considerable personal and political influence. If PHC professionals will eschew economic expediency and establish a disciplined integration of care and prevention, they could do much for world health by strengthening the resourcefulness and ability of the public to make more reasoned life-style choices for health and more political decisions which will aim at the kind of targets laid down for PHC at Alma-Ata (Appendix I).

References

Barr A, Logan RFL (1977) Policy alternatives for resource allocation. Lancet i:994–996

Bartlett EE (1980) The contributions of consumer health education to primary care practice: a review. Med Care XVIII, 8:862–871

Bax M, Hart H, Jenkins S (1980) The health needs of the pre-school child. Quoted in: Healthier children – thinking prevention (1982) Report of a Working Party. Royal College of Practitioners, London

Becker MH, Haefner DP, Kasl SV, Kirscht JP, Maiman LA, Rosenstock IM (1977) Selected psychosocial models and correlates of individual health-related behaviour. Med Care XV, 5:27–46

Becker MH, Maiman LA (1979) Patient perceptions and compliance: recent studies of the health belief model In: Haynes RB, Taylor DW, Sackett DL (eds) Compliance in health care. Johns Hopkins University Press, Baltimore

Berne E (1966) The games people play. Andre Deutsch, London

Black D (1980) Inequalities and health. Report of a DHSS Working Group. DHSS, London

Blaxter M (1981) The health of children. A review of research on the place of health in cycles of disadvantage. Heinemann Education, London, p 221

Breslow L, Enstrom JE (1980) Presistence of health habits and their relationship to mortality. Prev Med 9:469–483

British Nutrition Foundation (1975) Department of Health and Social Security and Health Education Council Working Party on Nutrition Education. DHSS, London

Church M (1979) Dietary factors in malnutrition: quality and quantity of diet in relation to child development. Proc Nutr Soc 38:41–49

Cleveland Health Education Department (1982) The health and health education needs of the inner city urban areas of Middlesbrough. Mimeo p 36. West Lane Hospital, Acklam Road, Middlesbrough, Cleveland

Cochrane AL, Holland WS (1971) Validation of screening procedures. Br Med Bull 27(1):1–8

Colver AF, Hutchinson AJ, Judson EC (1982) Promoting childrens home safety. Br Med J 285:1177–1180

Consultative Document (1976) Departments of Health in Great Britain and Northern Ireland. Prevention and health, everybody's business. HMSO, London

Curtis-Jenkins G (1980) The first year of life. Churchill Livingstone, Edinburgh

Department of Health and Social Security (1976) Fit for the future. The Report of the Committee on Child Health Services. Chairman SDM Court. HMSO, London

Durkheim E (1951) Suicide— study in sociology. Glencoe Press, New York

Edstrom K (1980) How can health services be made more relevant to the needs of mothers and children. In: Philpott RH (ed) Maternity services in the developing world. Proceedings of the Seventh Study Group of Royal College of Obstetricians and Gynaecologists. Royal College of Obstetricians and Gynaecologists, London, pp 351–359

Emery FE, Hilgendorf RL, Irving BL (1968) The psychological dynamics of smoking. Research Paper No. 10. Tobacco Research Council, London

Gatherer A, Parett J, Porter E, Vessey M (1974) Is health education effective? Monograph Services No. 2. Health Education Council, London

Hannay DR (1980) Religion and health. Soc Sci Med 14A:683–685

Harris DM, Guten S (1979) Health protective behaviour. An exploratory study. J Health Soc Behaviour 20:17–29

Hart JT (1975) Screening in primary care. In: Hart CR (ed) Screening in general practice. Churchill Livingstone, Edinburgh, pp 17–29

Hart JT (1980) Hypertension. Churchill Livingstone, Edinburgh

Hume Hall R (1974) Food for naught. The decline in nutrition. Harper and Row, New York London

Jelliffe D, Jelliffe E (1975) Human milk, nutrition and the world resource crisis. Sci NY 188:557–561

Journal of Clinical Nutrition (1953) Editorial. J Clin Nutr 1:149

Kingston P (1982) Power and influence in the environment of family therapy. J Fam Ther 4:211–227

Lalonde M (1974) A new perspective on the health of Canadians. Government of Canada, Ottawa

Langlie JK (1977) Social networks, health beliefs and preventive health behaviour. J Health Soc Behaviour 18:244–260

Leathar DS (1980) Images in health education advertising. Health Educ J 39(4):123–128

McLaren DS (1975) The great protein fiasco. Lancet ii:93–98

Marsh G, Kaim Caudle P (1976) Team care in general practice. Croom Helm, London

Mayer EE, Sainsbury P (1975) Promoting health in the human environment. WHO, Geneva

Meadows SR (1977) A developing specialty. Br Med J (Book Review) 1:1527–1528

Morrell D (1978) Screening in general practice. Health Trends 10:40–42

Newell KW (1975) Health by the people. WHO, Geneva

Passmore R, Hollingsworth DF, Robertson J (1979) Prescription for a better British diet. Br Med J 1:527–531

Pearce IH, Crocker LH (1944) The Peckham Experiment: a study in the living structure of society. George Allen & Unwin, London

Pill R, Stott NCH (1982) Concepts of illness causation and responsibility. Soc Sci Med 16:43–52

Rose G (1971) Early diagnosis of chronic disease. Br J Hosp Med 6:647

Rosenstock IM (1974) Health belief model and preventive health behaviour. Health Educ Mono 2(4):354, 2:328

Royal College of General Practitioners (1981) Health and prevention in primary care. Report from general practice, No. 18. Royal College of General Practitioners, London

Royal College of General Practitioners (1982) Healthier children — thinking prevention. Report of a working party. Royal College of General Practitioners, London

Russell MAH, Wilson C, Taylor C, Baker CD (1979) Effect of general practitioners' advice against smoking. Br Med J 2:231–235

Sackett DL, Holland WW (1975) Controversy in the detection of disease. Lancet ii:375

Schoenborn CA, Danchik KM (1980) Health practices among adults: United States 1977. Advance Data No. 64. Public Health Service, Washington DC

Scotney N (1980) What the community needs. In: Philpott RH (ed) Maternity service in the developing world. Proceedings of the Royal College of Obstetricians and Gynaecologists, London, pp 330–341

Scrimshaw NS (1964) Nutrition and stress. In: Diet and bodily constitution. CIBA Foundation Study Group, No. 17. Churchill Livingstone, Edinburgh, pp 40–48

Stacey M (1980) Realities for change in child health care: existing patterns and future possibilities. Br Med J 280:1512–1515

Stephen WJ (1981) An analysis of primary medical care: an international study. Cambridge University Press, London

Stott HH (1959) A pilot health study of the Zulu of Botha's Hill. PHA/33. WHO, Geneva

Stott HH (1973) African patients and nutrition education. In: Campbell GD, Seedat YK, Daynes G (eds) Clinical medicine in Africans in Southern Africa. Churchill Livingstone, Edinburgh, pp 502–506

Stott HH (1976) The Valley Trust socio-medical experiment in a less developed rural area. MD Thesis. University of Edinburgh, Edinburgh

Stott NCH (1981) Anticipatory care. In: Cormack J, Marinker M, Morrell D (eds) Teaching general practice. Kluwer, London, pp 193–197

Stott NCH, Pill R (1980) Health beliefs in an urban community. Report to DHSS. Department of General Practice, Welsh National School of Medicine

Task Force Report (1976) Preventive medicine. USA health promotion and consumer health education. Prodist, New York

The Valley Trust Annual Reports (1954–1982) Botha's Hill, Natal, South Africa

Tones BK (1979) Past achievement and future success. In: Sutherland I (ed) Health education: perspectives and choices. George Allen & Unwin, London, pp 240–262

US Departments of Agriculture and Health Education and Welfare (1980) Nutrition and your health. Washington DC

US Senate Select Committee on Nutrition and Human Needs (1978) Dietary goals for USA, 2nd edn. Washington DC

Van den Dool CWA (1970) Huisarts and Wetenschap 13:3 & 59. Mentioned in Hart JT (1975)

Vaux K (1976) Religion and health. Prev Med 5:522–536

Williams AF, Wechsler H (1972) Interrelationship of preventive actions in health and other areas. Health Ser Rep 87:969–976

Wilson JMG (1965) Some principles of early diagnosis and detection. In: Teeling Smith G (ed) Surveillances and early diagnosis in general practice. Office of Home Economics Press, London, pp 5–10

Yellowlees WW (1979) Ill fares the land. James Mackenzie Lecture 1978. J Roy Coll Gen Pract 29:7–21

Zinken PM, Cox CA (1976) Child health clinics and inverse care laws. Br Med J 2:411

6. The Refuge: Ethics, Practices and Problems

A "refuge", according to the New Oxford Dictionary, is a "place of shelter from pursuit, danger or trouble" and it can be a "person, a course or a thing that is resorted to in difficulties". From birth to death all people need periodic resort to a refuge while they shelter from life's trials and prepare to step out again into society. Sometimes home is a refuge, sometimes a friend, a spouse, the Church or one's God provides this function, but at other times distressing symptoms or fears drive people to medical services.

Those in caring professions are often thrust into the role of caring for refugees from distress and yet many great physicians of the past have taught their students to guard themselves against undue emotional sensitivity. Osler is reputed to have said "a certain measure of insensitivity is not only an advantage, but a positive necessity in the exercise of a calm judgment ...", and Brett Young commented on "the fallacy of medical callousness in relation to pain and distress ... if a doctor exaggerates the importance of subjective sensations in a patient he may lose sight of his own objective, which was nothing more or less than removing the cause". Kessel (1979) quoted both these great men but balanced their rather radical views of medicine in his fine essay on reassurance; he said:

> The doctor is required to stand apart. From his detachment, as much as from his knowledge, stems his authority and the ascendancy he must exercise over his patient. Patients are not everyday people but weakened people, who need the doctor to be a pillar of strength. He must respond appropriately. Medical men are often justifiably accused of treating patients too much like children or ignoramuses, but on the other hand patients are not normal strong adults. Critics of doctors forget that ill people may require to be dependent.

To be dependent is not, however, to be inferior or less able to take an informed interest in most decisions.

The mantle of authority which most doctors seem to adopt soon after qualification helps them to contain both the uncertainty and human frailty which they and their patients must feel on occasions, but this mantle also has disadvantages. First, it has been a cover from some ghastly and unjustifiable fashions in medicine, for example the removal of good teeth and organs in the pursuit of hypothetical "focal sepsis", or the exhibition of polypharmacy in the pursuit of pharmaceutical redress for every distress. Secondly, it has encouraged a dominant focus on physical procedures, drugs and organic interpretations at the relative cost of the complex dynamics of human relationships and the psychosocial antecedents of ill-health which come less readily under clinical manipulation. However, neither of these disadvantages removes the fact that when your child is ill, your mother dying or your wife is injured, a person needs comfort and reassurance and a feeling that something is being done. "Blind trust in the doctor", Bernard Shaw observed, "is the only practical alternative under such circumstances", but he was also scornful of the self-satisfied and pompous confidence which patients seem to have to accept as part of the healing package from some doctors. Shaw accepted his dependence on doctors and resented it.

In Table 6.1, an attempt has been made to portray, in as succinct a form as possible, the varied faces of clinical medicine from one extreme, of the unconscious patient who is in no position to exert personal choices and is totally dependent on the professional life-savers, to the opposite extreme, of the doctor who uses the clinical situation to encourage a desirable change of life-style, be it dietary or a habit. The need for a negotiating attitude increases

Table 6.1. The stratification of roles in medicine: management of need

Doctor–patient interaction

Doctor role	Patient role	Patients' needs
Active life-saver	**Passive**	Medical emergency Surgery
Director of therapy	**Collaboration**	Many conventional clinial problems
Supportive or **nondirective**	**Insight** and **adjustment**	Emotional problems Chronic disease Terminal care
Proposer	**Assessor**	Health education Prevention

progressively from the top to the bottom of the table and the dominating authority of doctors in an intensive-care situation becomes increasingly incongruous as the patient's perception of a problem becomes more of a force to influence the outcome and to interact with any clinical recommendations or proposals. The Bernard Shaw type of doctor is a colourful fragment of the true situation, but Shaw is right to tease doctors who have learned no other interpersonal skills except that of the authority figure.

An important prerequisite of reassurance is information about the condition in terms which are comprehensible and presented in a way which is likely to be believed, yet information sharing is often missing from consultations (Byrne and Long 1976) and all patients know that at the heart of the clinical encounter there are skills and attitudes which differentiate the doctor "who you can talk to" from the distant controller of a life-support machine or one who is (hopefully) better with his hands than with relationships (see Chap. 1). Both types of doctor, however, provide the patient wth a refuge at different levels of patient participation and both extremes are valued by the public for different reasons.

"Get me to the hospital" screamed the terrified victim of an assault which had left an arm bleeding and torn.

The public can be quite adamant when it is a technical approach to a problem that they want, but they can be equally confident when they are searching for understanding and information as well as clinical skill.

"You won't send me anywhere, will you doctor?" said the elderly man with a heart attack, who was living in a poor and grubby flat which had been his home for 30 years. "I know that you can help me and when the end eventually comes I want it to be here with my dogs and my memories of Sarah."

The synthesis of care and science is deeply entrenched in medical practice, yet there is evidence from many quarters that scientific structure and discipline can squeeze out the compassion which marks a refuge, and administrative efficiency can encourage the separation of caring and technical functions. The hospital bed which is emptied as quickly as possible to make room for "specialist material" leaves little room for its refuge functions, the out-patient clinic which is run like a production line leaves little room for its refuge functions, and the primary care clinic which processes patients so fast that they hardly have time to sit down may dispense medical provisions and technical help but is unlikely to provide more than a token refuge to people in distress.

Ethical and economic dilemmas surround how much clinical services should be involved in the provision of a refuge for distressed people rather than diseased people, and certain trends which have developed in British PHC illustrate this point.

Five Themes and an Ethical Dilemma

Five themes which have evolved in British PHC during the last decade are relevant to consideration of a refuge function.

1) A trend towards it being regarded as praiseworthy if PHC consultation rates and night-call rates are low. This should probably be dubbed the "John Fry theme" because he has publicised his evidence of low consulting rates in his British general practice (Fry 1972) and he is quoted by many other workers on this theme.

2) A trend towards refusing to prescribe for self-limiting minor ailments. This should probably be dubbed the "Geoffrey Marsh theme" because of his dramatic and publicised success at persuading his patients to accept their own responsibilities with regard to the management of minor ailments (Marsh 1977).

3) A trend towards anticipatory care in PHC which should be dubbed the "Van den Dool and Tudor Hart theme" because between them they have stimulated great interest in this approach to secondary prevention in cardiovascular and other disorders (Van den Dool 1975).

4) A trend towards teamwork in PHC which involves so many authors that it can only be dubbed the "management theme" (Pritchard 1978).

5) A fifth interesting trend is the goal of PHC for all by the year 2000 (see Appendix I). The "Year 2000 theme" has been kindled by the World Health

Organisation in the belief that PHC in some form should be available to all people. In this regard it is paradoxical that the British public was told that the National Health Service would look after them from cradle to grave yet by 1980 HM Government was saying that people really must do more to care for themselves.

Each of these themes deals with the issue of creating a society which has less need for curative medical services. The first by reducing demand, the second by reducing prescribing, the third by reducing the complications of ill-health, the fourth by using a team to do clinical work, and the fifth reflecting the paradox between WHO and British Government policies.

Interesting and important as each of these themes is, when considered together they represent quite a trend to imposed rationalisation of the use of PHC and a distinct shift towards separating patients from doctors and nurses. Some of the assumptions behind the drive towards separation certainly need to be highlighted and questioned.

Do we in PHC neglect the reasons for distress if we dwell too much on patient demand?
Do we in PHC worry more about drugs than the reasons why many people take them?
Does self-care really reduce demand for professional care?
Is PHC an arm of the state or a professionally disciplined system of personal care?
Is primary prevention a legitimate goal for PHC?

The first three questions provide a challenge to a trend in PHC which focuses on the surface features of work-load, drugs, etc. and neglects the fundamental reasons and mechanisms which underpin the operational surface. All three questions have been amplified in Chapter 4 and these will not be rehearsed; but the fourth and fifth challenges reflect the grey area between disease management and health promotion where special ethical and practical problems have been raised. The principle of opportunism which encourages doctors/nurses to use their clinical influence to encourage patients to reconsider their life-styles in the interests of future health has not been accepted unconditionally, and many critical comparisons have been drawn between the shift in governmental policy towards encouraging self-care and healthy habits and the stance being adopted by some clinicians who have shown that they have a role in health promotion as well as disease treatment. Social scientists have been particularly hostile to medicine's new roles and their views are of more than academic interest.

Holtzman (1979) has argued vigorously against the principle of prevention and health promotion through an emphasis on individual responsibility for life-style choices because he feels that such a policy will widen the disparity in health between the rich and the poor. He asserts that the most able will respond and the least able will lag behind and be condemned for their indolence and inept choices, and he states that "The doctrine of self-help may well signal a new era of Social Darwinism; those who cannot help themselves deserve their lot", and those who fail to conform to (medically) approved behaviour could stand condemned or victimised. An alarmist view was also stated by Crawford (1977) who coined the term "victim-blaming" to describe the consequences of a society which pursues health with such vigour that nonconformists become to be seen as outcasts and irresponsible. People who have lung cancer could be to blame because they smoked, those who are fat could become guilty of greed, those who have accidents may be negligent, those who are promiscuous deserve infertility. . . .

A shift away from the traditional nonmoralising stance of the trusted clinician could lead to serious changes in the doctor–patient relationship by introducing notions of blame for illness which are normally eschewed by the medical profession (Davis 1979). For example, the social condemnation of venereal disease has led to the development of confidential clinics and it is possible that the simplistic labelling of malnutrition, lung cancer, ischaemic heart disease, peptic ulcer, etc. as "diseases of life-style" could lead to difficulties in the provision of care for sensitive patients with these conditions. A doctor or nurse, who should be a neutral provider of refuge, may come to be perceived as one who is often judgemental about the style of life the patient has led, and therefore less sympathetic to current needs.

The Burning Question

The burning question for those in PHC is: can we provide care in the event of ill-health as well as negotiate with patients and others to prevent ill-health? Davis (1979) addresses this issue in his paper on "an unequivocal change of health care policy", which draws attention to problems over conventional medical models which, he alleges, preclude the development of alternatives to the clinical crisis orientation based on specific aetiology and specific therapy for an illness. He points to the asymmetry of the power relationship between the medical profession and society and describes angrily the inequalities of health care and medicalisation of everyday life, finally implying that a policy to encourage self-care and a preventive strategy which encourages people to reconsider their life-styles are nothing more than "an attempt to stem the rising tide of demand for health care by re-defining responsibility in illness". By shifting the blame for causation from the "external" factors (weather, climate, pollution, etc.) to "internal" factors (diet, smoking, promiscuity, etc.), Davis perceives that governments and the medical profession are locked in a mutually beneficial goal to control the volume of distress which people bring to the doctors' consulting rooms and yet to maintain a monopoly in matters of ill-health.

> If illness is the result of individual choices and not of "natural" processes, then to become sick is to be morally culpable . . . illness becomes a failure, a sanctuary is lost . . .

This slightly desperate yet persuasive idea is followed up at the end of the paper by a remarkable interpretation from another well-known social scientist:

Parson's characterisation of professionalism as affectively neutral, specific and technically efficient depicts a form of medical encounter which precludes doctors from intervening to change "life-styles" in a manner which is currently being suggested. Such a relationship has its benefits — in practice it limits medicine's involvement in everyday life, it eschews overt moralising, it also maintains a distinction between illness as a "natural" phenomenon as opposed to a "social" phenomenon.

It is vitally important for students of PHC to realise that the social scientists quoted here appear to have lost sight of the fact that medical knowledge about the causation of ill-health is changing rapidly. Fifty years ago many of the factors which are now causing the controversy about life-style and responsibility for health were not even recognised as serious threats to health, and it is extraordinary that critics of the integrating movement in PHC are striving to discourage clinicians from trying to carry preventive information to the most sensitised recipients: patients who are already seeking help from doctors or nurses or aides in or near their homes. These patients are often ready to hear or learn because they are worried about their health. Preventive information or help can be tailored to the individual's needs because of the one-to-one nature of most PHC contacts and the probability of involving the family in the decisions taken.

Critics of the integration of prevention and cure in clinical medicine are often unwilling to accept that it is possible to provide therapy in the event of illness and to care enough to try to prevent disease; that it is possible to have encouraged or helped a smoker to give up his habit and still have a supportive and understanding relationship when he develops lung cancer some years later; that failed contraception is not always seen by clinicians as being due to carelessness; that the causes of obesity do not need to be thrust at the hapless sufferers from the complications of obesity; that learning how to reduce the risks of malnutrition or any other illness does not provide a guarantee for future health because social forces can operate to undermine the resilience of the most health-minded person. In other words, responsibility for personal health or ill-health is at best partial because of the complexity of the issues, and blame is seldom valid or humane. A clinician who condemns people for their styles of life is unlikely to be competent as a carer or as provider of a refuge when illness really strikes.

The Refuge Role in Clinical Practice

Medicine grew in stature as a refuge long before modern cures and modern knowledge became available, and the credibility of the physician/nurse still hinges on an ability to provide a refuge.

A primary refuge from distressing symptoms and from fear of serious disease has been offered by clinicians for centuries as they provide reassurance, symptom relief and cures.

A secondary refuge when "official" sanction of the sick role is required by society (certification) to provide proof of bona fide illness which prevents patients from fulfilling their social functions.

A tertiary refuge when the distressed and/or diseased person needs hospital care, a hospice or a place of safety for healing, relief or protection.

Most human health problems are still self-limiting if the individual can be sheltered temporarily from continuing stresses and nourished appropriately; like a wounded animal, we seek a safe shelter while the body heals and then embark once more on daily life. Even the exacerbations of chronic disease often respond more to rest than to therapy, so over the years "masterly inactivity" has become a respectable clinical strategy.

The modern interventionist approach to illness and to health promotion/prevention has sometimes overshadowed the older refuge which is only tacitly accepted in many quarters despite the glaring evidence for its continuing importance. For example:

Most acute illness is self-limiting — yet many people continue to need a healer for reassurance and explanation when they become anxious about the possibility of more serious things.

Many acute specialist hosital beds are used for either refuge or temporary hostel functions (Farrer-Brown 1959; Department of Health and Social Security 1971).

A very high proportion of hospital out-patients does not require the highly specialised facilities associated with district general hospitals in most parts of the world (King 1966; Wade and Elmes 1969; Department of Health and Social Security 1971; Gruer 1972; Lindgren 1973).

The community-based peripheral clinic with very basic and simple facilities is being recognised as an essential resource in both developed (Gruer 1972) and less developed (King 1966) areas of the world (Lindgren 1973; Sai 1973) because specialised or complex interventions are not necessary in the majority of problems.

Care of the dying has been bedevilled by an attitude of technical defeat — "nothing more I can do" — just when the patient and family need a refuge most for relief, for security and for hope. The growth of a "hospice movement" has been necessary to highlight this blindness (Saunders 1978; Wilkes 1980) and to shame doctors and nurses into recognising that when nothing more curative or technical is available, they continue to carry a responsibility to offer dying patients a refuge of primary, secondary or tertiary type.

It is no accident that the first cottage hospital in Britain in 1858 was described by its founder as "literally a cottage, with an optimum of six to eight beds, differing only from patients' homes in cleanliness, warmth, proper hygiene and absence of overcrowding" (Napper 1979). The first cottage hospital was provided by the benefactors and people of a district and no doubt they, the providers of a little refuge, had some influence over its use as a local amenity.

As specialist medicine grows and blossoms in its curative glory, the basic human need for a refuge has not changed but the willingness to honour that need is not always clearly visible. This can be well illustrated by considering how the tertiary institutional refuge has become progressively more technical in its functions and more aggressively rehabilitative in its goals.

Local nursing homes and small community hospitals are easily squeezed out by more expensive and specialised central hospitals (Fig. 6.1). The patient who needs only rest, nutrition, nursing and reassurance for healing to occur does not always find that such simple, yet fundamental facilities are available. The gap between home and hospital is sometimes so wide that the compassionate clinician is unable to provide for an obvious need — the temporary institutional refuge. It is as if many planners are blind to the reality of the temporarily dependent patient and they devalue the need for a continuum of refuge facilities from the primary ambulant to the tertiary bed-bound. Instead of a continuum of facilities, we often find a staggering gap into which fall the unfortunates who are too distressed to be left at home yet too well to be in a specialist hospital bed. Primary health care still holds a key to many refuge needs because it deals more in distress than in disease, and more in pain than in wounds (see Chap. 4). Our credibility with patients often hinges more on our compassion and our willingness to provide a temporary refuge in a crisis than on major diagnosis or treatments.

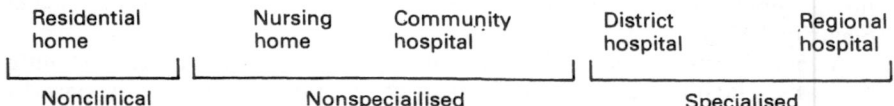

Fig. 6.1. The spectrum of institutional care — the refuge of those who cannot be at home. Do you have a full range in your area?

Brimblecombe (1979) re-discovered this basic truth when he investigated the needs of families with a handicapped child. As a good paediatrician, he was sensitive to family feelings and he found that they were describing to him well-documented PHC concepts.

1) Families need continuity of care from a professional person who has access to the necessary knowledge and develops a genuine personal relationship with the family so real communication can occur.
2) Families need to achieve independence and self-reliance by acquiring the essential skills, confidence and courage needed to help (the child) achieve full personal potential.
3) Families need most support in times of crisis or difficulty so they do not feel isolated and get exhausted or bitter.

All three needs are highlighted in handicap, but those with experience in PHC will recognise that the first is the primary or secondary refuge, the second a statement of the principles described in Chapter 4, and the third the tertiary refuge. Brimblecombe discovered for handicapped children a series of PHC principles which apply to greater or lesser extent to the population at large; principles which a general paediatrician was able to identify and understand as well as a good general practitioner but which many specialist colleagues have considerable difficulty in grasping.

100

The Temporarily Dependent Patient

The concept of the temporarily dependent patient (Thomas 1974) is close to the heart of good general clinical practice in most cultures because it has a connotation of caring without encouraging unnecessary dependence and even without always formulating a diagnosis or therapy (other than reassurance). For example, K. B. Thomas collected a series of patients in British general practice who had consulted with nonspecific, probably self-limiting problems (40% of the patients seen in 45 surgery sessions) and allocated them randomly to two groups.

Half were given symptomatic diagnoses and treatment.
Half were simply given reassurance that they had no evidence of disease.

No significant difference was found in the outcome of these two groups as judged by return to normal, complications and satisfaction with the consultation (Thomas 1978), suggesting that contact with the family doctor was sufficient and neither his prescriptions nor his words of reassurance were as important as his confidence in the outcome of each illness. Was the doctor a drug? (Balint 1975). One suspects not, because confidence is built on trust and trust cannot be dispensed like a drug, it must have been earned before the trial was started and occurred equally in both groups of patients studied.

Whatever clinicians do in terms of trying to encourage a change of habits, or acceptance of therapy, or reassurance, or referral, or monitoring, or modification of expectations, or health education — each can only be successful if the patient feels that the professional helper is willing to provide specific technical care when it is necessary and equally willing to provide temporary refuge when that is appropriate.

The International Discipline of Primary Health Care

As PHC becomes recognised as an international discipline, there is a grave danger that it will either become fragmented and distorted into its component technical parts (as many specialists would like to see) or practised in a rigid way with the doctor or nurse imposing an intellectual agenda too firmly on every situation. The framework in this book is an aide-memoire to the surface anatomy of the potential in each consultation; it is not the agenda for every consultation because often it is wholly inappropriate to widen the consultation beyond a sensitive response of the presenting distress. A grief-stricken or anxious person has no motivation to modify a destructive life-style and someone in physical pain will be most concerned with quick relief. However, the search for meanings and interpretation will follow as pain and distress come under control and then unique opportunities arise for widening the consultation potential to embrace much more than the immediate felt needs.

Those who are prepared to provide a refuge hold a key to public confidence and nowhere is this truth more evident than in the doctor or nurse or aide with a willingness to integrate the intellectual agenda of PHC with the crisis needs of patients and their families.

Successful negotiation for health can only occur within a context of mutual respect, respect that is earned by responding sensitively to crises which are brought to primary health care (Periera Gray 1977), and by providing the resulting sensitised person(s) with practical and personal help rather than general woolly advice. Once the refuge has sensitised the person, opportunism in health matters can often flourish (Fig. 6.2) and the process of negotiation with the individual/family can begin on a level and at a pace compatible with their needs and abilities.

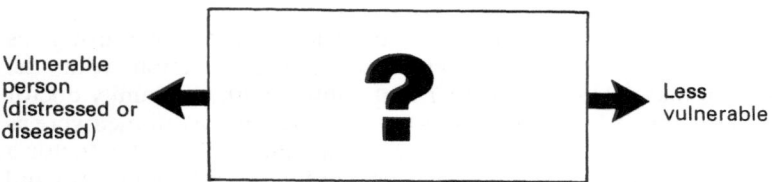

Fig. 6.2. The clinical process(?) which provides opportunities for cures, for care and for the promotion of more health-giving life-styles.

The importance of the refuge function in PHC is often implied rather than stated in clinical texts which dwell only on the availability, accessibility, economy and morbid content of PHC. Diseases occur in people and sometimes diseases are preventable by individual actions, but neither disease management nor preventive activity is likely to be adopted unless there is confidence in the humanity of the carers. "Can you help doctor(?) or will you try to manipulate my disease or my way of life before you have even offered me a refuge in distress?" The refuge is one key to credibility in PHC and without it we can only be technicians with limited goals or frustrated professionals who lack the resources to provide more than specialised fragments of PHC.

The clinician who keeps the surface anatomy of PHC in mind on the daily round is unlikely to become so fascinated by one part that sight is lost of the rest. Specialists should indulge in fragmented fascinations but generalists dare not lose sight of the totality of their discipline or they will simply slide into becoming specialists. The aide-memoire to the anatomy, physiology and pathology of PHC described in this book is offered as an aid to keeping our discipline on target as we go about our daily work.

References

Balint M (1975) The doctor, his patient and the illness. Pitman Medical, London

Brimblecombe SW (1979) A new approach to the care of handicapped children. J Roy Coll Phys Lond 13(4):231–236

Byrne P, Long B (1976) Doctors talking to patients. A study of the verbal behaviour of general practitioners consulting in their surgeries. HMSO, London

Crawford R (1977) You are dangerous to your health: the ideology and politics of victim blaming. Int J Health Services 7(4):663–679

Davis AG (1979) An unequivocal change of policy: prevention, health and medical sociology. Soc Sci Med 13A:129–137

Department of Health and Social Security (1971) The organisation of group practice. Chairman R. Harvard Davis. HMSO, London, p 68

Farrer-Brown L (1959) Hospitals for today and tomorrow. Br Med J 1:188–192

Fry J (1972) Twenty-one years of general practice — changing patterns. J Roy Coll Gen Pract 22:521–528

Gruer R (1972) Outpatient services in the Scottish Border Counties. Scottish Health Service Studies, No. 23. Scottish Home and Health Department, Edinburgh

Holtzman NA (1979) Prevention: rhetoric and reality. Int J Health Services 9(1):25–39

Kessel N (1979) Reassurance. Lancet i:1128–1133

King M (1966) Medical care in developing countries. Oxford University Press, London, pp 3.11–3.15

Lindgren SA (1973) Sweden. In: Douglas-Wilson I, McLachlan G (eds) Health service prospects. The Lancet Publications, London, pp 99–123

Marsh G (1977) "Curing" minor illness in general practice. Br Med J 2:1267–1269

Napper A (1979) Quoted by Loudon ISL. The general practitioner and the hospital. In: Fry J (ed) Trends in general practice. Royal College of General Practitioners, London, p 99

Periera Gray DJ (1977) General practitioners and the independent contractor status. J Roy Coll Gen Pract 27:750–756

Pritchard P (1978) Manual of primary health care: its nature and organisation. Oxford University Press, London

Sai FT (1973) Ghana. In: Douglas-Wilson I, McLachlan G (eds) Health service prospects. The Lancet Publications, London, pp 125–155

Saunders C (1978) Hospice care. Am J Med 65:726–728

Thomas KB (1974) The temporarily dependent patient. Br Med J 1:626

Thomas KB (1978) The consultation and the therapeutic illusion. Br Med J 1:1327–1328

Van den Dool CWA (1975) Quoted by Hart JT. Screening in primary care. In: Hart CR (ed) Screening in general practice. Churchill Livingstone, Edinburgh, pp 17–29

Wade OL, Elmes PC (1969) An analysis of out-patient referrals. Update June:721–724

Wilkes F (1980) Terminal care — report of a national working group. Standing Medical Advisory Committee. HMSO, London

Appendix I Declaration of Alma-Ata

The International Conference on Primary Health Care, held in September in Alma-Ata, the capital of the Soviet Republic of Kazakstan, expressed the need for urgent action by all governments, all health and development workers, and the world community to protect and promote the health of all the people of the world. The following declaration was pronounced.

I

The Conference strongly reaffirms that health, which is a state of complete physical, mental, and social wellbeing, and not merely the absence of disease or infirmity, is a fundamental human right and that the attainment of the highest possible level of health is a most important worldwide social goal whose realisation requires the action of many other social and economic sectors in addition to the health sector.

II

The existing gross inequality in the health status of the people particularly between developed and developing countries as well as within countries is politically, socially, and economically unacceptable and is, therefore, of common concern to all countries.

III

Economic and social development, based on a New International Economic Order, is of basic importance to the fullest attainment of health for all and to the reduction of the gap between the health status of the developing and developed countries. The promotion and protection of the health of the people is essential to sustained economic and social development and contributes to a better quality of life and to world peace.

IV

The people have the right and duty to participate individually and collectively in the planning and implementation of their health care.

V

Governments have a responsibility for the health of their people which can be fulfilled only by the provision of adequate health and social measures. A main social target of governments, international organisations, and the whole world community in the coming decades should be the attainment of all peoples of the world by the year 2000 of a level of health that will permit them to lead a socially and economically productive life. Primary health care is the key to attaining this target as part of development in the spirit of social justice.

VI

Primary health care is essential health care based on practical, scientifically sound, and socially acceptable methods and technology made universally accessible to individuals and families in the community through their full participation and at a cost that the community and country can afford to maintain at every stage of their development in the spirit of self-reliance and self-determination. It forms an integral part both of the country's health system, of which it is the central function and main focus, and of the overall social and economic development of the community. It is the first level of contact of individuals, the family, and community with the national health system bringing health care as close as possible to where people live and work, and constitutes the first element of a continuing health care process.

VII

Primary health care:

1. reflects and evolves from the economic conditions and socio cultural and political characteristics of the country and its communities and is based on the application of the relevant results of social, biomedical, and health-service research and public-health experience;
2. addresses the main health problems in the community, providing promotive, preventive, curative, and rehabilitative services accordingly;
3. includes at least: education concerning prevailing health problems and the methods of preventing and controlling them; promotion of food supply and proper nutrition, an adequate supply of safe water and basic sanitation; maternal and child health care, including family planning; immunisation against the major infectious diseases; prevention and control of locally endemic diseases; appropriate treatment of common diseases and injuries; and provision of essential drugs;
4. involves, in addition to the health sector, all related sectors and aspects of national and community development, in particular agriculture, animal husbandry, food, industry, education, housing, public works, communications, and other sectors; and demands the coordinated efforts of all those sectors;
5. requires and promotes maximum community and individual self-reliance and participation in the planning, organisation, operation, and control of primary health care, making fullest use of local, national, and other available resources; and to this end develops through appropriate education the ability of communities to participate;
6. should be sustained by integrated, functional, and mutually supportive referral systems, leading to the progressive improvement of comprehensive health care for all, and giving priority to those most in need;
7. relies, at local and referral levels, on health workers, including physicians, nurses, midwives, auxiliaries, and community workers as applicable, as well as traditional practitioners as needed, suitably trained socially and technically to work as a health team and to respond to the expressed health needs of the community.

VIII

All governments should formulate national policies, strategies, and plans of action to launch and sustain primary health care as part of a comprehensive national health system and in coordination with other sectors. To this end, it will be necessary to exercise political will, to mobilise the country's resources and to use available external resources rationally.

IX

All countries should cooperate in a spirit of partnership and service to ensure primary health care for all people since the attainment of health by people in any one country directly concerns and benefits every other country. In this context the joint W.H.O/UNICEF report on primary health care constitutes a solid basis for the further development and operation of primary health care throughout the world.

X

An acceptable level of health for all the people of the world by the year 2000 can be attained through a fuller and better use of the world's resources, a considerable part of which is now spent on armaments and military conflicts. A genuine policy of independence, peace, détente, and disarmament could and should release additional resources that could well be devoted to peaceful aims and in particular to the acceleration of social and economic development of which primary health care, as an essential part, should be allotted its proper share.

The International Conference on Primary Health Care calls for urgent and effective national and international action to develop and implement primary health care throughout the world and particularly in developing countries in a spirit of technical cooperation and in keeping with a New International Economic Order. It urges governments, W.H.O. and UNICEF, and other international organisations, as well as multilateral and bilateral agencies, non-governmental organisations, funding agencies, all health workers, and the whole world community to support national and international commitment to primary health care and to channel increased technical and financial support to it, particularly in developing countries. The Conference calls on all the aforementioned to collaborate in introducing, developing, and maintaining primary health care in accordance with the spirit and content of this Declaration.

Appendix II Hand-out for Clinical Tutors in Primary Health Care*

The Teaching of Medical Students in PHC

Clinical Sessions with Tutors

The overall aim of undergraduate teaching in PHC is to provide teaching and learning opportunities for students in those aspects of clinical medicine which are most satisfactorily studied in the community or practice setting, thus complementing experience in other clinical specialties. It also offers a continuing opportunity to develop basic clinical skills. Students are expected to become familiar with the wide potential in every consultation. Hence continuing clinical problems, help-seeking behaviour and opportunistic health care will receive appropriate consideration in all patients.

Tutors are involved mainly with clinical teaching and each student will go to a clinical tutor for at least x half days over a period of y weeks.

The precise allocation of the students' time with their tutor will be at the discretion of the tutor. The following, however, may help you in devising a programme.

1) We want students to learn by "doing", hence the student need not be with you all the time. We imagine that the student will, on each morning or afternoon spent with you, sit in on a consultation session with you. During the remainder of that morning or afternoon students can usefully:
   i) go on visits with you,
   ii) go on visits to selected patients on their own,
   iii) visit the patient whom you have selected as the subject of the case study which we require them to undertake.

2) We believe that students will learn most by being as involved as possible in patient care. To this end, we suggest that students can be given patients with chronic problems or thick case notes to visit, and make a summary and suggest a plan of management which may be of value to the practice.

The following outline is intended to help you to introduce some structure to the consulting session in your own clinical teaching, BUT PLEASE REMEMBER THAT THE BEST TEACHING WILL ALWAYS focus on what is available at the time.

*Hand-out for clinical tutors receiving medical students during their final year of training at the Welsh National School of Medicine.

107

Session	Core theme
1 Orientation	General orientation to the practice and how a consulting session functions. Student(s) will probably watch you at work and should begin to feel that they can recognise some problems. Suggest that the student makes a note of the problems with which he/she is (1) familiar, (2) unfamiliar. This can aid discussion. Please emphasise aims for the NEXT session *before* students leave you.

2 & 3
Presenting and
   continuing problems
	The students should be making diagnoses and suggesting treatment for common presenting problems, e.g. upper respiratory infection, otitis media, tonsillitis, cystitis, diarrhoea and vomiting, trauma, social discord, etc. Please make them consult while you watch for at least a couple of patients during the session and teach on (1) skills — especially ENT examination, (2) choice of treatment — especially the reasons why you choose what you prescribe, (3) what proportion of patients come for diagnosis or reassurance rather than treatment, (4) the "ticket phenomenon" (e.g. child presented with coryza when mother really wanted to discuss fertility).
	   NB The students are taught to avoid broad-spectrum antibiotics in sore throats and tonsillitis and to avoid antimicrobial therapy for most diarrhoeal illnesses. They may be unaware of the difficulty over accurate diagnosis of UTI before treatment in the community. The value of health visitor and social worker in management will also be new.
	   Please also comment upon the CONTINUING problems your patients have (even if they have chosen to ignore them), e.g. a woman with a flu-like illness *may* have a past history of recurrent UTI or obesity or irregular menstruation, etc. Doctors frequently assess such things to check that the problem(s) is resolving, but students may not realise that you are practising "continuing care" unless you are explicit. If your clinical records do not communicate continuing problems clearly, please *discuss* this with the students so they realise *why* the records don't help and how they could assist in continuing care if differently organised.
	   Finally, please mention aims of fourth sessions to students.

4
Opportunistic
   care and
   anticipatory care
	By now the students should be comfortable with you and capable of assessing common problems with minimal help. They should also be looking for continuing problems in patients which merit monitoring or a follow-up check.
	Now introduce the more controversial idea of PREVENTIVE care in selected patients. The students should be able to identify two broad areas where

108

preventive intervention could be to the patient's benefit:
1) Where early diagnosis is desirable,
     e.g. has blood pressure been checked within 5 years?
          eyesight in elderly with family history of
          glaucoma?
          squint in infancy?
          growth in socially deprived child?
          routine MSU after recurrent urinary infection?
          cervical cytology?
2) Where life-style choices are important,
     e.g. smoking habits
          abuse of alcohol
          poor dietary habits
          use of drugs in pregnancy
          accidents in the home
          immunisation
          relationship conflicts.

No general practitioner will/should deal with all possible
aspects at every consultation, but please try to
demonstrate awareness of looking at chosen patients in
this way. If you feel uncertain about the value of advice,
please discuss *why*, and point out that other methods of
health education are available to you: health visitor
groups, displays in waiting room, antenatal clinics,
media, etc. Also you will probably feel that your own
results are better with some aspects than others — help
the students to discover why this is happening.

5
Help seeking

In the final sessions we hope that the student will see
some patients alone (if you can arrange this) and that
you will emphasise how management modifies future
expectations.
     This may involve a problem of whether a particular
person should or should not be classified as "sick"; the
dangers of a "pill for every ill" or the use of repeat
prescribing or contraceptive services or immunisation.
In each situation the patient has to decide to seek help.
Whether the decision is appropriate or inappropriate
will be influenced by a consistent practice policy and
organisation over a period of time.
     What patients experience in clinic today may modify
what they expect tomorrow — for better and for worse.

Please remember the following topics are particularly relevant to undergraduates in *any* of the clinical sessions.

The infectious diseases.
The appropriate use of investigations.
Infant-feeding problems.
Immunisation decisions and problems.
Recurrent abdominal pain.
Catarrhal or atopic children.
Behaviour problems of childhood.

By the time the student leaves you he/she should have begun to see the importance of looking beyond the patient's presenting problems. But the potential and the barriers to achieving excellent continuing care and opportunistic care will have been discussed and health behaviour will have been considered – at least in so far as it has an impact on primary health care.

THANK YOU

Subject Index

111

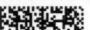